YOGA FOR WEIGHT LOSS

CELIA HAWE

Photography by Francesca Yorke

Kyle Cathie Limited

First published in Great Britain in 2003
under the title *Yoga for Slimmers* by
Kyle Cathie Limited
23 Howland Street
London W1T 4AY
www.kylecathie.com

This edition published in Great Britain in 2011

ISBN 978 0 85783 014 2

Text © 2003 Celia Hawe
Special photography © 2003 Francesca Yorke
Except pages: 21, 34-35 (centre), 54-55 (centre), 76,
77, 79, 94-95 (centre), 101, 104, 134 and 137; all by
Photodisc.

Project editor: Sarah Epton
Copy editor: Catherine Blake
Editorial assistant: Vicki Murrell
Food stylist: Annie Rigg
Designer: Becky Willis
Production by Sha Huxtable and Claudia Varosio

Celia Hawe is hereby identified as the author of this
work in accordance with Section 77 of the Copyright,
Designs and Patents Act 1988.

A CIP catalogue record for this book is available from
the British Library.

Colour separations by Scanhouse, Malaysia
Printed and bound in China by C&C Offset Printing
Company Ltd

Author Acknowledgements.

First and foremost, thanks to my beloved husband,
Peter, for his unending support, coaching and
enthusiasm, and for his input and work into the Yoga
for Weight Loss programme – and this book. Thanks
also to all the wonderful teachers, seminars, lectures
and books that have helped me along the way.
Writing this would have been impossible without
them all.

Grateful thanks must go to my publisher, Kyle Cathie,
editor Sarah Epton, designer Becky Willis,
photographer Francesca Yorke and food stylist Annie
Rigg. And not forgetting my beautiful yoga models
Juliet Murrell, Lisa Frize and Nicky Smith. Also Jenny
Pretor-Pinney for the use of her yoga studio
(www.yogaplace.co.uk), and Alice Asquith and Casall
(see Resources, page 140) for supplying the clothes.

Finally, on a personal note, thanks to my connection
with my own body, mind and spirit – a connection
which has pulled me through many a challenge over
the years and has enabled me to help and support
others through theirs.

Contents

Introduction

Yoga for Weight Loss is a fabulous, unique programme to help you become slim in body, mind and spirit. It is deliciously straightforward and contains a simple and easy routine, with lots of motivation and encouragement added in to support you. I'm convinced from my own experience, and from the results achieved by those who have followed the programme, that it is the only way to approach the 'dis-ease' – the discomfort and distress – of being overweight. In the 20 plus years I have spent studying yoga and working in the fitness industry, I've coached many thousands of people, helping them to lose fat and to learn to love themselves, and through this book I can now help you too.

Slimming from the inside out

According to popular belief, 'at my age' I'm supposed to be getting bigger around the middle and putting on weight. I promise you, this has not happened (well, I always was one to go against convention!). Since I've changed my mind set about being overweight with this winning yogic programme, I've stopped the endless cycle of weight gain and weight loss. It has put me back in control, and it can do the same for you. Together we will streamline your body by revitalising sluggish hormones and boosting your metabolism through incredibly powerful breathing techniques. Most important of all, I will teach you how to achieve awareness – your key weapon when you're fighting the flab. Through the positive, 'in control' approach that yoga inspires my attitude towards my weight has changed completely. I feel so proud to have lost so much weight and kept slim afterwards, whereas previously I berated myself for constantly oscillating between weight gain and weight loss.

I will also help you to look at things from a different perspective, and see that it is not a crime to be a little on the heavy side. After all, it's a great place to start! What if, just what if,

> My Yoga for Weight Loss programme will help you to lose fat effortlessly and permanently.
>
> All you have to do is:
> 1. A few easy postures
> 2. Challenge your present thinking
> 3. Follow an easy detox eating plan
>
> It works because:
> 1. It alters your way of thinking
> 2. It identifies areas of your life that need to 'lose weight'
> 3. The eating plan is practical, easy-to-follow and guarantees results

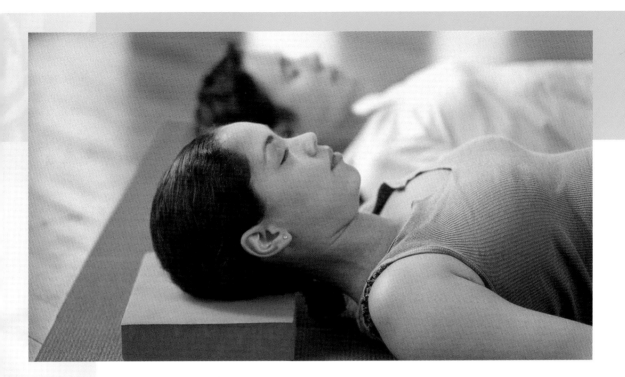

our bodies were exactly the size they were meant to be, so that, for some reason, we could learn a certain lesson by being overweight? Being overweight in today's society is seen as a failure. But what if you could see it as a message that you are living life out of balance? The important thing to remember is that being overweight is a symptom of a much greater malaise. Diets and strict exercise can, for a short time, admirably address the symptom of being overweight but, sadly, they often stop working, or we get bored, lose momentum or resolve, and give up, and then we perpetuate the hated cycle of feeling a failure, getting fatter and losing sight of the fact that we have to heal our whole self.

As I write this, I know that a large proportion of the population is suffering from the symptom of being overweight. So if being overweight is the symptom, what is the

disease? I believe that our lives are truly out of balance, that we have lost sight of our true nature; we are merely living to survive life and have forgotten how to achieve our full potential, how to be the joyous, loving, caring, radiant beings that we are. So if we could we tap into our true, authentic selves, reconnect with that part of us, our unnecessary fat would disappear. In order to do this, we need to develop the ability to empower ourselves to create the life we should be living. In case you are confused, or if no one has ever said anything like this to you before, let me repeat it: our unwanted fat is the symptom of a deeper disease, that of being disconnected from our true selves — our authentic humanity, which is loving, caring, kind, creative, and wise. If we can connect to this, then not only will we as individuals enjoy a wonderful life which at last makes sense, but also humankind as a whole will be uplifted. So, in this context, isn't it great that your body is giving you a message and thus the opportunity to raise your life to a higher level?

Yoga for Weight Loss will coach and motivate you to take time each day to reconnect with your deeper self. At first you will need to trust in the fact that it exists, so that you can strive for the connection. You will have to take my word for it that this will work. All I'm asking for is one month of 40 minutes a day to try it out. It's a small wager when the winnings are a totally new, slimmer, happier you. We will use simple postures and breathing techniques to give us space from our ludicrously artificially filled lives and allow this connection to take place — to realign ourselves. There are no complicated postures, there will be nothing asked of you which will be too arduous — unless you find slowing down difficult, and you probably will, to begin with. The benefits of taking time out will prove invaluable, and by simply committing to reconnecting to the wonderful you each day, you will magically find your whole life revolutionized. I know you only bought this book to lose a bit of weight, but think of it as a fabulous bonus! Anyway — as I always tell my yoga classes — don't believe a word I say, try it out for yourselves.

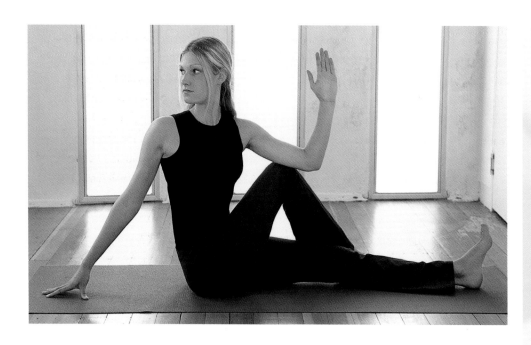

Time for some positive thinking

Let me be your own personal coach and yoga teacher. Imagine me there with you – talk to me, shout at me, whatever helps. But trust me: with this programme you will learn to love yourself instead of being full of fear. I know that fear attracts fat and if you are afraid of being overweight then inevitably you will seem to draw to you what you most dread. I also have found that a negative attitude towards yourself – loathing or chastising yourself as you may well be right now – also seems to slow down the slimming process. So even if you have to pretend to like yourself at the moment, do it!

Yoga also helps you develop your will-power; many wonderful women that I have coached told me that they had none, and felt desperate. Often these same women have achieved amazing things in their lives that required a lot of dedication, but have fallen by the wayside when it came to sticking to an eating regime. With this winning yogic programme you will restore your strength of will in every area of your life, and that is what it takes for you to exercise total freedom of choice and awareness in your life – forever.

You will also find that you get your body back into alignment. Even if you have a difficult day and you perform the exercises without any awareness at all, perhaps thinking about what you will cook for dinner or whether you should redecorate the living room, you will find that somehow you will tap into the 'energy' of the previous sessions and still derive great benefits. Of course, I would prefer it if you used your awareness to be present fully during the sessions so that you will make the most of the experience, but at whatever level you practise you will still get a lot out of it. Most of all, don't worry, because yoga is not about tying you in knots but helping to unknot you!

So commit to working through the book, with me, and you will become so much stronger, and gain a completely different perspective on life and your challenges. If I can do it, so can you.

Why me?

This is where I hope you will recognise that this book is for you, because the reason I wrote it was to share with others all the changes that yoga has brought into my life, particularly in controlling my weight. I know that all the ideas here will support you as you come to terms with being overweight, and how you look and feel in the world. I know how it feels because for most of my adult life I have considered myself overweight. And sometimes I was overweight. I blamed it on various sources – food manufacturers, my husband, my father, my mother, dinner parties, holidays, Christmas. Even throughout my years as a fitness centre owner, when I exercised regularly, I still felt fat. And so, it seemed, did everybody else. I interviewed and worked with thousands of women, and only one, in all the years I have been in the industry, has been pleased with her body. During all this time I was practising yoga and teaching it, but somehow it was separate from my fitness programme. It seemed to me that, wonderful as the yogic teachings were, they were devised more than 5,000 years ago by people whose lives were totally different from our own today. They didn't have an abundance of junk food, chocolate and alcohol to tempt them, nor were they leading the stressful and sedentary lives that blight so many of us now. But then I began to devote a lot more time to personal development, and spent weekends and vacations, time and money, visiting the USA and elsewhere to study and integrate yoga into my life as a fitness instructor.

Then, at the height of my career, when I was traveling around the world teaching, I developed Chronic Fatigue Syndrome. Although at the time this was a critical blow because I could no longer continue to teach exercise or run my classes, through being ill I was given more time to think, connect and listen. I listened to women and how they were reacting to their bodies, and I tried to make them laugh. But there was a serious intention behind my jokes — I wanted to help them see their weight in less threatening terms.

It pays to remember that the body believes every word we tell it at some deep, subconscious level, and it must be very demoralised when all it hears is how much we hate our shape and wish it were different. Through my illness, I was given the time to listen to myself and what my body, mind and spirit were trying to tell me, and I learned that communication is vitally important. That's why you will find a chapter on positive, accurate dialogue between your body, mind and spirit, and how crucial this is to support you in your programme to rid yourself of weight challenges.

As a consequence of my illness, I found I had to put myself together again, and out of this desire to get fit and healthy came a unique formula, my Yoga for Weight Loss programme. I already understood that yoga is one of the oldest exercise systems in the world and has huge health benefits physically, emotionally, and mentally. So the yoga, the personal development, my exercise expertise and my health awareness, born from my illness, all went into the pot. I took everything I already knew and developed a unique combination of exercises and nutritional, mental and spiritual support programmes to help me feel more alive and full of energy. A huge, unexpected bonus was that it also helped me to lose weight. This regime not only will slim you down and make you feel more vital than you have in years but also will help you to live at your full potential on all levels. It certainly worked for me: despite the increasing years I feel younger, more positive and more in control than I ever have in my whole life. Here are just a few of the things you will learn:

- How 'thinking big' is essential to weight loss
- How to boost your metabolism and lose weight
- How fear attracts fat
- How to fill your life with things you truly value
- How to make your mind work for you, not against you
- The power of loving and forgiving
- The secrets of breath control, to change your brain chemistry and soothe and balance you
- Meditation, visualisation and relaxation for weight control

My unique Yoga for Weight Loss programme has three steps:

Step 1 Learn all the postures outlined in chapters 3 to 10 and perform all of them, including the warm-up, meditation, and relaxation, daily.
Step 2 Complete the complementary personal development exercises.
Step 3 Follow the 28-day detox and eating plan.

My unique body-mind-spirit approach will help you lose fat and keep it off forever. Now, isn't that worth a month's dedication? With this book, you can realise the perfect you. So what are we waiting for?

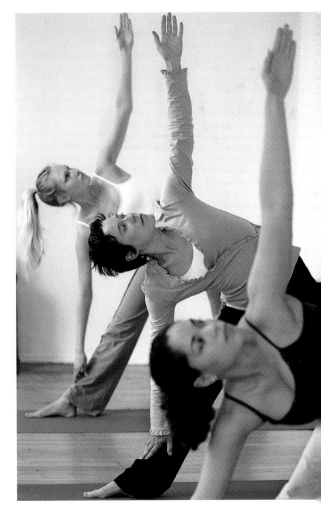

1 What is Yoga?

It is not essential to know anything about the history of yoga to practise it, but many people do like to learn more about where it came from and exactly what it involves. The actual word means 'union'. We join our 'little' self, known in Sanskrit as Atman, with our 'larger' self, or Brahman. Now, you are probably saying, what on earth is she on about? I don't want to join with any larger self, I want to be slim! Hang on. Traditionally yoga teaches that we each have a spiritual dimension that we can tap into, and in this way we transcend the body. With the Yoga for Slimmers programme, therefore, you engage with a philosophy in which ultimately it ceases to matter what size you are!

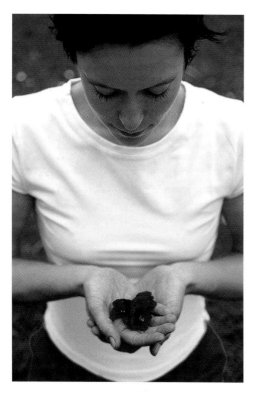

This may sound contradictory but the truth is that we can only challenge our size and shape successfully once we have embarked upon our journey towards this ultimate union. In fact, it's the ONLY way to lose weight permanently, because if there are no permanent shifts in your thinking then dieting will merely reduce weight temporarily. Dieting is like cutting down the weeds in your garden and expecting them never to grow again. If you don't want weeds, you have to pull them out by their roots. Yoga for Slimming is all about getting at the roots. Put another way, those reasons for your being overweight are fed by your 'little' self, and the more you move towards the 'bigger' self, the less power the little self will have over you.

It is hard to define yoga, since it can be many things to many people, but here are a few facts and perceptions:

■ Yoga is a very ancient practice that originated in India about 6,000 years ago. It consists of physical and mental disciplines that make us healthy, alert and receptive, transforming our perception of the world and the way we live in it. It allows the individual to achieve his or her full potential and then to stretch beyond into spiritual consciousness.

■ The word 'yoga' means 'union' or 'to yoke', implying the harnessing of oneself to a way of life as well as the union of all things. Yoga can be used at any level of living and can be adjusted to suit any daily routine.

■ Yoga can be looked upon as a technique of personal development that existed long before any system of philosophy. The *Bhagavad-Gita*, one of the principal sacred Hindu scriptures, describes yoga as:

■ equilibrium in success and failure
■ skilful living
■ the supreme secret of life
■ source of the greatest happiness
■ effected by self-control
■ non-attachment
■ the elimination of pain
■ serenity

■ Yoga produces an incredible feeling of joy, peace and beauty that is beyond words.

■ The yoga postures (*asana*) exercise every part of the body, stretching and toning the muscles and joints, the spine and entire skeletal system. They work not only on the body's frame, but also on the internal organs, glands and nerves, keeping all systems in radiant health. By releasing physical and mental tension they liberate vast resources of energy. The breathing revitalises your body and helps to control the mind, leaving you calm and refreshed, while the meditation gives you increased clarity, mental power and concentration.

■ Yoga subtly changes your approach to life; you begin to glimpse a state of inner peace which is your true nature.

■ Yoga is known to improve overall health and builds resistance to disease.

Yoga has been practised for thousands of years. It is a system of bodily and mental exercises whose aim is freedom. Physically it promotes stability, energy, flexibility and relaxation. Mentally it promotes concentration, balance and tranquillity. You learn to do the postures not by striving for perfection but by learning to let go of the stiffness and tensions that inhibit movement. Each stretch is a way of freeing your body from stress. The purpose of the postures is to readjust and realign your body to bring back its natural balance, by freeing the habitual blocks and tensions acquired over the years.

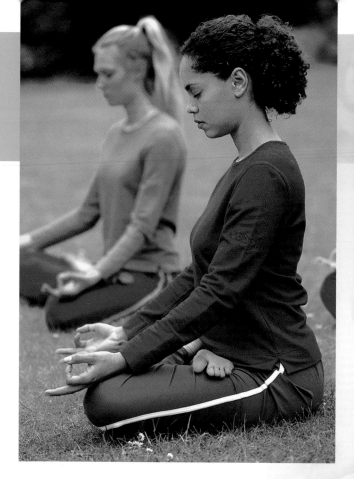

The value of yoga

Over the thousands of years that yoga has been practised there have been many claims made for it. It is widely accepted that yoga can to help you:

- Lose weight – either generally or in specific areas of the body.
- Improve your figure.
- Strengthen and recondition your entire body.
- Learn how to relax properly.
- Stay relaxed under pressure.
- Remove mental strain and tension.
- Improve your concentration.
- Become more sensually aware of yourself and others.
- Improve your circulation and breathing.
- Rid yourself of back problems.
- Get relief from conditions such as insomnia, headache, migraine, sinusitis and asthma.
- Improve the condition of your skin, eyes and hair.
- Eliminate many causes of depression.
- Regain agility and youth.
- Make sense of life.
- Experience a sense of oneness with yourself and others.
- Accept yourself just as you are rather than chastising yourself for not having the 'perfect' figure.
- Develop self-empowerment.

- Become more peaceful, individually and globally.
- Achieve the integration of body, mind and spirit so that you can live and act in harmony with all life.

Is yoga a religion? No, definitely not, but it is spiritual. That's why people from all religious persuasions, as well as atheists, use yoga. It can help deepen your understanding of your own particular religion or it can give you a fresh spiritual perspective on life. Or, you can just use the postures to help you achieve a more flexible body and clearer mind. You decide what you want from it. You set your goals and yoga will help you attain them.

The stages of yoga and how they help you

The yogis identified eight steps along the path to the state of total well-being. Yoga for Weight Loss works with most of these stages and also with different types of yoga. In fact, you could say that Yoga for Weight Loss is 'Fusion Yoga', which makes it sound very trendy! Yoga is not dogmatic – you just do your best. Sometimes we fall by the wayside but, as the song says, we just 'pick ourselves up, dust ourselves off, and start all over again'.

1. Yama

Yama is the firm determination to do something positive about one's life. It is about inner discipline and responsibility. Surely this is what we are doing by affirming our intentions to become slimmer, happier, healthier. *Yama* is about ensuring that we are not false or greedy, but live our lives in a way that causes no harm to ourselves or others. This includes animals, and that's why many yoga practitioners do not eat meat. Rejecting falsehood and greed is certainly good advice when it comes to slimming. I have frequently raided the fridge in the night, somehow kidding myself that since it's so late the extra food won't count. When we are miserable, unhealthy and not achieving our potential, we are harming ourselves. So *Yama* is

definitely a good discipline to adopt, and will help us through the programme.

2. Niyama

Niyama are observances, things we need to adhere to. These are purity, contentment, study, devotion. Purity and cleanliness are key values, both physically and mentally.

3. Asana

These are the postures that we perform in our yoga sessions. The aim is to achieve an effortless awareness in which the body is perfectly steady and relaxed. This is great, because through this awareness we will find it so much easier to keep to our programme. Such a lot in our world today is distracting us from everyday moment-to-moment awareness: noise, bustle, TV, crowded places. To learn to centre ourselves in the moment and be detached from all that is very helpful and something you will find beneficial in every area of your life for the rest of your life.

4. Pranayama

Pranayama is the control of *prana*, which is a life force within the body known as *chi* in Chinese medicine. We do this with our breathing exercises. The ancient yogis believed that there are 72,000 *nadis* or energy channels in the body – similar to those an acupuncturist uses – and by breathing in controlled ways we can help to energise and remove blocks in these pathways. Removing congestion in this way will support our endeavours to be lean and healthy.

5. Pratyhara

Withdrawal. This is the ability to withdraw our senses and remain unaffected by disturbances. Emotions, fears and the turmoil of modern living pull us away from our awareness of our deeper self, tempting us to comfort ourselves with food and drink, but through *pratyhara* we can overcome this. It strengthens our resolve, and is therefore self-empowering.

6. Dharana

Concentration. We practise and improve this by focusing on an object or name as we do in our mantra meditation. When I concentrate totally on something, I do not think of anything else, and that includes food.

7. Dhyana

Meditation. In meditation you try to become one with the object of your thoughts. So if you meditate on, say, a beautiful rose coming into blossom, and become one with that image, it will be reflected back in a 'blossoming out' of your life.

8. Samadhi

Enlightenment. You understand yourself and what life is all about. You no longer need to work hard at being a good, loving person because you just are like that. You have seen the reality of it all and realise that we are all one, therefore you do not want to harm another person; in fact you do not have to try to love anything, because you become love itself. At this level you will experience bliss, true bliss – and it has nothing whatever to do with fattening food!

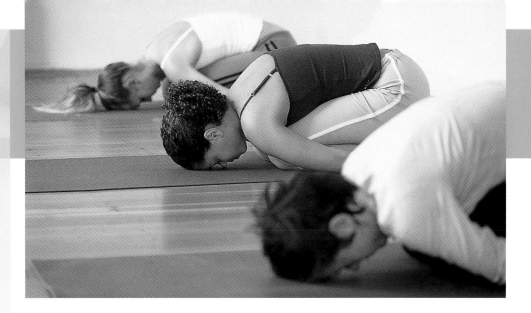

The paths of yoga

Hatha yoga

This is the physical yoga intended to balance and harmonise your body so that you can reach and manifest your full potential. In this instance, of course, we want to achieve slim, lean, healthy bodies – which is actually our natural state of being. Hatha yoga puts the responsibility for your health and well-being firmly into your own hands.

Karma yoga

The yoga of action. It teaches you to sublimate the ego, and therefore to act selflessly, without thought of gain and reward.

Bhakti yoga

The path of devotion, which includes prayer, worship and ritual. This yoga surrenders to God and unconditional love. Often chanting is used to sing the praises of God, and this forms a substantial part of Bhakti yoga.

Jnana yoga

The yoga of knowledge and wisdom. You use your mind to inquire into its own nature. This is considered the most difficult yogic path.

Raja yoga

This is the science of physical and mental control. It puts you in charge of the waves of your thoughts by turning your mental and physical energy into spiritual energy.

So that's yoga summed up very simply and briefly. You can mix and match the different types of yoga to get a designer-made system just perfect for you. I've developed the Yoga for Weight Loss programme in this way, so that it's right for your needs. I hope I've whetted your appetite and you are eager for second helpings! There are many excellent books around on yoga, so get studying because it's a fascinating, self-empowering subject, which can help you make sense of your life and live it to its full potential (without the added calories).

Guidelines for Successful Practice

Yoga for Weight Loss is a safe, health-promoting programme which has been specially designed for people who are new to yoga as well as those of us who are overweight.

However, if you have any serious health problem or are very overweight, consult your doctor before starting the programme. This is a good idea anyway if you are over 40 years old and have never exercised before. Many doctors are aware of the benefits of yoga and frequently recommend it for people who are suffering from the effects of stress, tension and a host of other ailments. If you have specific health challenges at the moment, it may be necessary to avoid some of the postures, and also to proceed with caution, especially to begin with. Just check through the following list so that you know how best to proceed.

You are undertaking a very personal programme, and are not in competition with anyone, not even yourself. The programme should be approached VERY GENTLY to begin with. The number of repetitions or the time spent on the postures should be increased very slowly and gradually.

Please remember that progress is faster when you take it slowly. This may seem a

■ If you have heart disease or high blood pressure, a detached retina, weak eye capillaries or problems with your ears that could be exacerbated by extra pressure, are pregnant or menstruating, do not do the shoulder stand; just lie with your feet up against the wall.

■ If you have arthritis, be gentle with yourself until you find out what works best for you. You may need to adapt a posture, use cushions, or hold on to something to support you.

■ If your back is vulnerable, be careful when you do the back bends. Start gently and you will find that, along with the other postures, they will aid the recovery of your back by improving the tone and flexibility of surrounding muscle tissue.

■ During menstruation, avoid the shoulder stand. Also be gentle pulling the abdominal muscles in and out when you perform the yogic tummy tuck.

■ If you have a contraceptive IUD fitted, do not perform the yogic tummy tuck too strenuously, for you could dislodge it.

■ If you have high blood pressure, you need to be careful with breath retention. Retain the breath for only a very short period — if at all.

contradiction, but it is absolutely true. Never force any movement – yoga is intended to 'unknot' you, not tie you up in knots. I usually start the postures with my right side first but you may start with whichever side feels more comfortable and then repeat on the other side. Your body's wisdom is an excellent teacher and yoga will help you develop the awareness necessary to access it.

Focusing on the benefits

To get the most out of anything we undertake, I believe we need to understand fully why we are doing it and how it can help us. Throughout the following chapters, key words are given to describe the benefits each posture provides in terms of body, mind and spirit.

The mind and spirit key words can also be used as affirmations or focus points as you perform each posture. You are free to decide, according to your present needs, whether you would benefit by focusing more on the key words for the mind, strengthening your intention, or on the spiritual dimension of the practice.

This radical approach, encompassing the mind and spirit in exercise, might feel strange at first, but the results will astound you. Why limit the benefits of the postures to just the physical? It can be the icing on the cake – and unlike the other kind, it helps you actually lose weight!

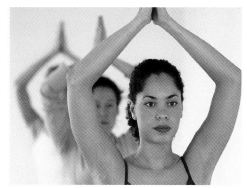

Body

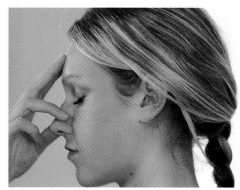

Mind

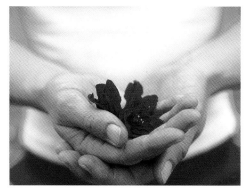

Spirit

Here's your initial checklist to get you started on successful yoga practice:

■ Put aside specific times in your day to enjoy your practice. This time is special, like making a date with yourself, but a very special part of yourself. This is the 'higher' part of you that is always there, but you must learn how to connect to it.

■ Avoid exercising on a full stomach; allow 3–4 hours after a meal or 1 hour after a snack.

■ Take a bath or shower beforehand, if you can.

■ Turn the phone off, and hang a note on the door to say that you are having time to yourself. This is YOUR time.

■ Leave all your concerns, excitements and worries outside the door.

■ Wear light, loose clothing, preferably made of natural fibres, that does not restrict your movement and that you feel comfortable in. Keep these clothes especially for your session. Have your feet bare.

■ In the morning or during cold weather your muscles will be stiffer, so ease carefully into the postures at first.

■ Perform all the postures slowly and with control, concentrating on your breathing and relaxing into the positions. Let go of any unnecessary tension and maintain an uplifted feeling in body and mind.

■ Hold the postures for approximately 20–30 seconds, breathing normally – that is about 4–7 breaths. Hold for a shorter time if you are out of condition and not used to exercise, or for a little longer if you wish.

■ Once is sufficient for each posture but you can perform it 2 or 3 times if you wish. However, remember that it is more important to maintain regularity of practice because you will get more benefit from having shorter, more frequent sessions than sporadic lengthy ones.

■ Begin each posture with great awareness, hold with great awareness, and come out with great awareness.

■ Learn the exercises, or postures, by working with the book to begin with and then use the quick-reference guide to the postures (see page 143) to prompt you.

■ Get a special yoga mat for yourself. This is really important, not just because it makes your practice easier and safer, but because this is your sacred space or temple (or whatever you wish to call it). It is just for you, so don't let anyone else step on it or use it, because you will eventually build up energy on your mat that will support you throughout the programme. Of course the height of luxury would be a room set aside as a special place, but failing that your special mat is your portable temple!

And finally, a question of attitude

Over the years of teaching yoga, I have noticed that how you approach your yoga is usually how you approach life. Think about it. Do any of these statements apply to you?

- Do you approach your yoga by trying to get it over with as quickly as possible?
- Do you give up, complaining that it's all too hard?
- Do you miss important bits out?
- Is your mind filled with 'to dos'?
- Do you feel selfish or guilty for taking time for yourself?

This simple assessment of your attitude to your yoga practice can help you make adjustments that will produce permanent benefits in all areas of your life – and this is just the beginning.

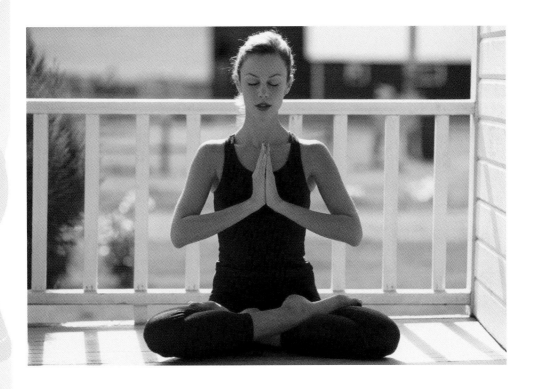

3 Let's Begin: The Essential Warm-up

So now you are ready to begin your Yoga for Weight Loss practice, and the starting point is always to get the body warmed up and ready. It is a very important part of the regime and, just to remind you, you are going to perform each posture once and hold it for approximately 20–30 seconds, breathing normally. This is usually about 4–7 breaths, but do it within a shorter time if you are out of condition and not used to exercise. Remember that because these exercises are all part of your warm-up you will not hold these stretches as long as you would the postures in the main body of our session.

Attunement

This is the key to your getting limbered up and becoming focused prior to the session proper, so don't miss this out. No matter how busy or short of time you may be, it's crucial that you do this every time since it will prime your body to get the most out of your session.

■ Physically these light movements ensure that synovial fluid lubricates the joints and that chemicals in the muscles are 'switched on' and alerted for more dynamic stretches.

■ Mentally the attunement ensures that you are fully present for the postures.

■ Spiritually it prepares a sacred space in readiness for you to connect with your deeper self – if you like, symbolically putting on your spiritual robes.

Let's start.

Focus to start – letting go

■ Lie down flat on your mat to start your session. Begin by thinking of that special place inside you where you know you are perfect, and try to visualise it. Envisage yourself moving into it. You are connecting with your true self, the perfect part that exists and that is a true reflection of how special you are. Is that new to you, the idea that there is a part of you that is so special? Well, it's true, but you will just have to take my word for it to begin with. This special place we invoke at the start of your session is best described as a place of alert stillness.

■ As you lie on your mat, let go of any tensions, excitements, problems and concerns, so you are relaxed and focused. If you find this difficult, you can imagine that there is a wooden chest outside the door; see yourself opening the lid and putting these problems, excitements and worries into the container and shutting the lid. They are going to stay there until you decide to let them out. During the time that you are practising your yoga they are safely contained and won't bother you.

Breathing to Start – Calming Breath

To start your yoga time you need to be in a place of calmness, and calming breath can help you to get there. This is a very balancing and healing breath. It is a way of tuning into your body's wisdom: it knows what you need, and it helps prepare you for your yoga session. You can also use it to calm and re-balance yourself at any time when you might be feeling stressed or pressured. For pictures, see over the page.

1 Lie flat on your back, feet about 45cm (18in) apart, toes relaxing outwards, hands away from the body with the palms uppermost. I call this the Rejuvenation Posture. If it is uncomfortable for you to lie flat, you can bend your knees and put your feet flat on the floor. You may also like to support your head using a standard-size telephone directory (if you don't have a yoga block), or a cushion of similar thickness, which helps to lengthen the neck (see picture 1a). Again, this will suit some people but not others, so experiment to find what is best for you.

2 On your in-breath make sure you breathe right down into your lower abdomen. If it helps, put your hand there for the first few breaths – you will notice that your hand rises slightly.

■ Breathe in and sigh the breath out. Feel the whole of the back of your body in contact with the ground.

■ Very simply – just breathe in for a count of 2, hold the breath for a count of 2, breathe out for 2 and hold that out-breath for 2. Do this a few times and, after a while, when you've become comfortable with the rhythm, let the counting go. Breathe in, pause and just hold the pause until the body decides it wants to breathe out, and then breathe out, and let the pause on the out-breath happen naturally. This completes one full cycle. Do 7 more cycles of this breath. Always finish on the pause after the exhalation to complete the breathing cycle.

■ Work slowly up to a pattern of 10:5:10:5 – breathe in for a count of 10, hold for a count of 5, breathe out for a count of 10, and hold the out-breath for 5. This is the yogic breath that optimises your metabolism.

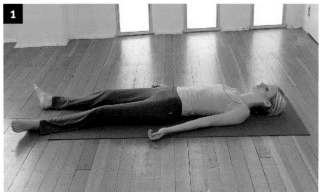

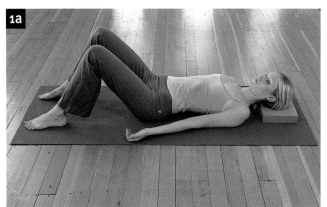

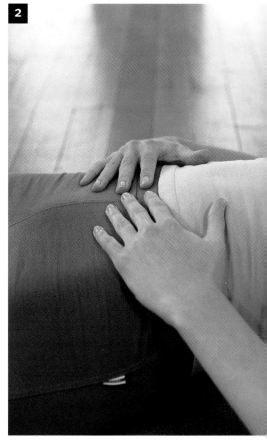

TIP – You can also use this breath to give you a strong focus. For instance, if you are having a difficult day with your slimming programme and your will-power is low, you could use it this way: breathe in will-power, on the pause say to yourself, 'I bathe my whole body in will-power,' then, as you breathe out, breathe out anything that is getting in the way of your will-power. Then, on the holding-out pause, you say, 'I am full of willpower – now.' This is a very simple but also very powerful technique, and you can use it to help you whenever you need support.

Full Body Stretch

Perform the movements with a sense of pleasure, anticipation and openness, and any tension will just drop away. Let your breathing stay relaxed and natural, and while you practise these movements see yourself as you want to be. Picture yourself moving through life at your correct weight. Bring to mind the emotion that you feel. What is it you really want to achieve? How will your life be different? Remember this feeling as you do this full body stretch.

1 Lying flat on your back, extend your arms beyond your head, resting them on the floor, and, with your legs outstretched flat, breathe in and stretch from your fingertips to your heels. Exhale and relax.

■ Keeping your arms overhead, stretch the right side on an inhalation; exhale and relax.

■ Now stretch the left side as you breathe in, and then exhale and relax. Your left arm is still on the floor beside your head, stretching away.

■ Then stretch the right arm and left leg as you breathe in; exhale and relax.

■ Then stretch the left arm, which is still behind you on the floor, and with it your right leg as you breathe in, then exhale and relax.

■ Now stretch from your waist upwards as you breathe in, and then exhale and relax.

■ Finish by stretching everything below the waist; flex the feet and push the heels away as you breathe in, and then exhale and relax.

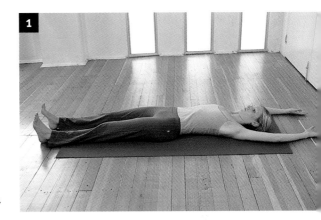

TIP – This may not be easy at first, so spend some time co-ordinating your movements and your breath until it feels natural. You are learning to relax the different parts of your body individually. This will be crucial to you in your weight-loss programme because stress and tiredness often lead to overeating as a way of trying to get more energy into the body. When you are stressed, the muscles tense up, which is a waste of your body's energy. So you need to learn how to relax at will and become much more aware of your body – techniques that will help you achieve the body you desire.

Knees to Chest

Keep your head relaxed, using a yoga block, telephone directory or cushion for support if you need it. Notice any stiffness and encourage your body to let it go by mentally relaxing that area. Bring to mind a feeling or quality that you need or would like to have more of today, such as joy, abundance, prosperity, peace, clarity – choose one or more.

1 Begin by lying on the floor, hands by your side with your knees bent on to your chest and your feet hip-distance apart.

2 Rub your hands together very quickly and imagine putting your chosen quality into your palms.

3 When your palms are really hot, put them over your knees and let this quality permeate into your knees.

■ Keep your hands where they are. Imagine this quality going down right to your toes.

■ Now visualise it travelling up your body to your head and brain.

■ Then imagine it going down your shoulders and back down your arms to your hands.

■ If you wish, you can radiate this quality out a few centimetres away from your body so that you are 'cocooned' in it.

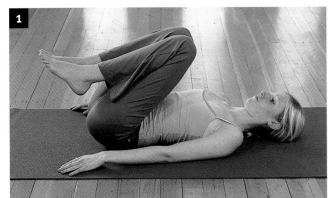

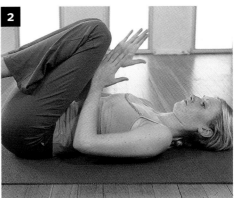

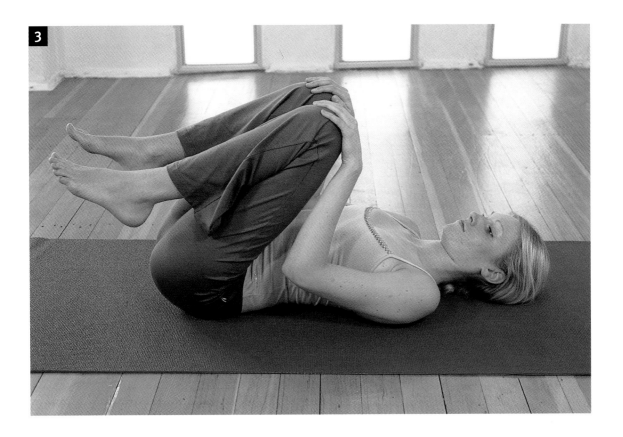

Knee Circles and Side-to-side

1 Keeping your hands on your knees, make small circles with them – 7 times in a clockwise direction and 7 anti-clockwise. Keep your knees together and the rest of your body relaxed, so you are giving your lower back a good massage on the floor. Try to keep your shoulders and back flat on the floor.

2 Take your knees about 35cm (14in) apart and slowly lower them to one side, taking your head in the opposite direction. Let your elbows stop you going over completely. Repeat on the other side. Do this 4 times each side.

3 Bring your knees back to the centre and lower both legs down flat on to the ground. Rest the arms.

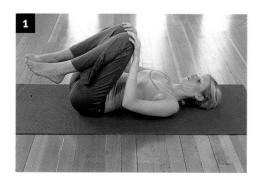

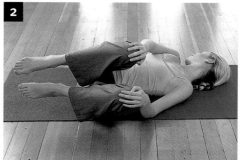

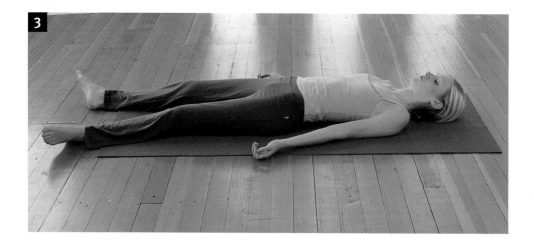

Hip Loosener

1 Clasp your hands around your right shin and gently bring your right knee into your chest. Make sure that you never put any pressure on your knee caps. Extend your left leg straight on to the ground. Hold for a few seconds and enjoy the stretch.

2 Now take your right knee out to the right side, keeping your left buttock firmly on the ground so that your hips stay level. Rest your hand on the inner thigh. Hold this position for a few seconds, feel the stretch in the groin area

and relax into it. You can use your right hand to press gently down on your right leg, easing it down to the side, but remember not to press on the knee itself.

3 Now take your right knee across to the left side, performing a gentle, limbering spinal twist. Extend your right arm out to the side at shoulder height.

■ Turn your head to face your right arm, so that you are looking in the opposite direction to your knee. You may use your left hand to ease the knee gently into a comfortable stretch.

■ Bring the knees back to the centre, and straighten the right leg. Repeat the Hip Loosener on the other side.

4 Come up to a standing position by curling up and rolling on to your right side, taking 2 deep breaths, and gradually coming upright. Remember that going into and out of the postures is an important part of the practice, so don't rush it. Try to add a sense of focus and higher awareness to your movements as you do this.

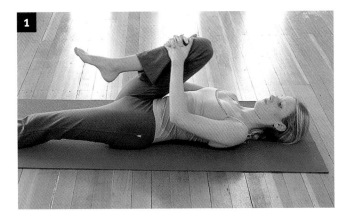

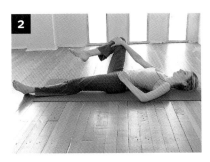

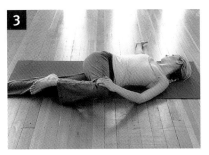

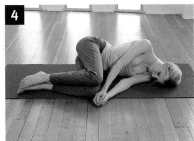

Poise

The simplest way to lose 2kg (5lb) – and look younger – is to stand correctly. This posture helps release upper-back tension. Body and mind are totally integrated, so an uplifted body leads to an uplifted mind. Slouching is depleting, your back muscles and the functioning of your abdominal organs are affected, breathing is impaired and your digestion is also impeded.

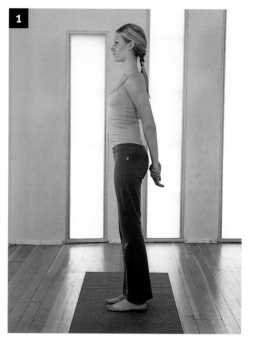

1 Stand comfortably with the feet parallel and shoulder-width apart. With the right middle finger and thumb, encircle the left wrist behind your back (see picture 1a) and gently extend your arms downwards.

■ Notice how your posture immediately improves and your chest expands, making breathing deeper and more efficient (remember, oxygen is necessary for optimum metabolising to help burn fat more quickly). Feel the stretch in the front of your shoulders. Ease your shoulders back and down, and lift your head up, keeping your chin parallel to the floor. Notice how this posture uplifts your spirit. You will feel better and stronger, and more determined to stick to your Yoga for Weight Loss programme.

■ Hold this for 3 deep breaths and repeat, holding the opposite wrist.

TIP – Do this any time during the day to help energise you and correct any energy-depleting body posture.

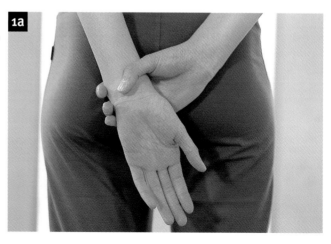

Mountain (Tadasana)

You will use this position often in your yoga practice.

1 Stand upright with your feet comfortably together or slightly apart but parallel and flat on the floor, hands by your sides.

■ Allow your body to stretch naturally and extend upwards as though you have a knot of hair on top of your head which is being gently pulled up, but keep your chin parallel to the floor. Notice the slight tension in the buttock and abdominal muscles, keeping the body upright. Attempt to lift yourself 2 or 3cm (1in) taller.

■ Feel equal weight on each foot; make any small adjustments to bring this into being. Have approximately two thirds of your weight on the balls of your feet and one third on your heels.

■ Notice how by standing correctly you feel stronger and more aligned in your body. This will help you visualise how your body and mind are interconnected and therefore how important the postures will be for your psychological as well as your physical well-being.

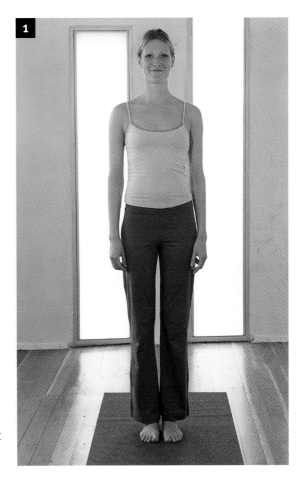

4 Success: The Choice is Yours

In this chapter we are going to look at the quality of the choices you are currently making, and at how you can learn to strengthen what I call your 'choice muscles'. To lose fat your choice muscles must be effective for all your waking hours, and this takes energy – any less than this and your old, unsupportive thinking and behavioural habits automatically take over. So to lose weight successfully you need to free up energy, both physically and mentally, to provide the fuel to keep your goals alive.

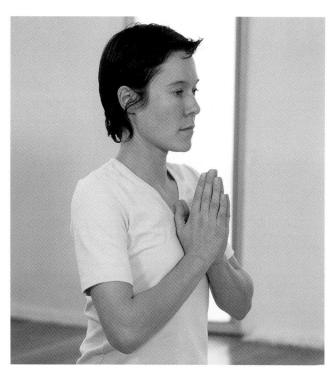

Making healthy choices

At the risk of upsetting or angering you, how would you feel if I asked you to accept that you are overweight because at some level you choose to be? Whatever your immediate response to that statement may be, would you be willing just to sit with it and observe what is happening to you as you think about its implications? If you can begin to accept it, it will take you from being a victim to being empowered. Then you can start to make the choices in life that WILL make you slim.

When I was overweight I believed I had no choice: I felt compelled to eat, and to satisfy myself with food. It was as though biscuits in a tin were tied together and magnetically found their way to my mouth. At the time it didn't seem as if I had any time to make a decision, because those biscuits just disappeared so quickly! But if you start to realise that you are not a victim, and that you really can decide what and how you eat, then you will succeed.

I think that coming from this perspective of choice is extremely important and that is why I ask you to exercise your choice muscles with each posture. When the time comes for you to move out of a posture, I ask that you make a choice, whether to stay where you are, to come out, or to go a little deeper for a few seconds – or you can at any time choose not to do that posture and just lie or sit still.

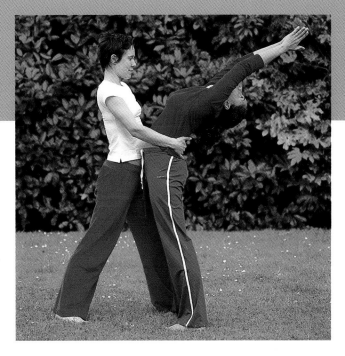

Training those choice muscles is a wonderful preparation for day-to-day living, especially where food is concerned. I can't emphasise strongly enough that you really do decide what you eat, and that decision has consequences. If you choose a healthy, low-fat, low-sugar meal, the payoff will be that you will lose excess fat and achieve a slim body. If you choose to eat high-fat junk food then, for sure, you will retain fat on your body and your weight will increase as a result of this. Fact – although many times I've kidded myself this was not so – the choice *is* yours.

Setting successful goals

Before any journey we need to set some basic goals. As the old adage goes, 'If you don't know where you are going, you'll never get there.' We need to set some basic goals to point us in the right direction. It's my belief that we often inadvertently set ourselves up for failure when we choose our slimming goals. Here are two that I've struggled with, and I expect you have suffered similarly. First goal: 'I will lose 1kg [2lb] per week.' To set yourself such a goal is unfair on yourself, since the goalposts keep moving. Fluctuations in weight may have nothing to do with fat but with some other factor, such as the amount of fluid in the body. Fluid retention can be caused by the onset of menstruation, for example, or salt intake. So you may actually

have worked hard and lost body fat, but end up weighing more by the end of the week. The second goal that caused me problems was this: 'I will lose 1 stone by my birthday.' This one caused me so much stress that I inevitably failed. Like the unfortunate Sisyphus of Greek legend, I was condemning myself to push a heavy rock uphill over and over to reach a goalless goal. Then I felt miserable, put on more weight and entrapped myself in a vicious circle.

I also believe that if you give yourself an unattainable goal your subconscious mind cannot assimilate it and therefore does not help you to achieve it. For instance, many diet programmes advocate sticking up a photograph of someone whose body you wish yours could look like, in a place where it might prove a timely reminder, such as the fridge door. But you are not Julia Roberts or Kate Moss, and never can be. Similarly, fear tactics don't work either. The ploy suggested here is usually to put a photo of you at your fattest on the fridge door to deter you from snacking or overeating. All this does is breed negativity. Your mind can be your greatest friend or your greatest enemy, and you need it to work with you, not against you. So think carefully about the type of goal you are setting yourself.

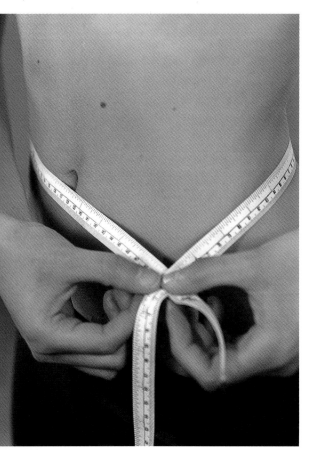

Smart goals

To set your Yoga for Weight Loss goal we need to work with the SMART method of goal setting, which has proved highly effective. SMART goals are Specific, Measurable, Attainable, Realistic and Time-framed.

Complete the following:

My Yoga for Weight Loss goal is to

....

I will have achieved this by

....

I know I will have achieved it because I will

....

and feel

....

or be able to

....

Here is an example of how this works:

My Yoga for Weight Loss goal is to
read this book
....
I will have achieved this by
next week
....
I know I will have achieved it because I will
understand the empowering message this book has for me
....
and feel
inspired
....

Is this SMART? Yes, it is SPECIFIC because there is the book to read, it's MEASURABLE because there are a certain number of pages, it's ATTAINABLE because I know I can read a book in this time, it's REALISTIC because it's a straightforward and easy book to read and it's TIME-FRAMED because it's to be done by next week.

A not-so-SMART (but maybe more familiar) goal might be:

My Yoga for Weight Loss goal is to
lose 5kg (11lb)
....
I will have achieved this by
2 weeks
....
I know I will have achieved it because I will
weigh in on my bathroom scales 5kg lighter
....
and feel
great
....

Is this SMART? It's specific and measurable, but not necessarily attainable because weight loss depends on so many other factors outside your control. If you want your goals to be smart they have to follow the SMART rules. Read the book and forget about setting weight loss goals. You will come across more tips about goal-setting, on pages 78–79.

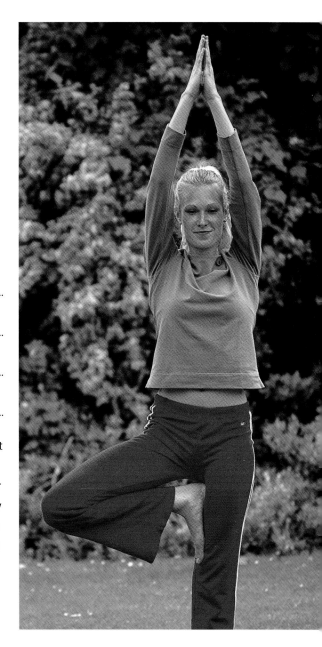

Finding the energy to lose weight

As I've said before, to achieve your goals you will need energy. One way to free up more energy is to block any energy leaks. I call them 'energy bandits' because they steal your time and focus, and allow your energy just to seep away. If you find this hard to imagine then try this little experiment. Get a paper or plastic cup, think of something that irritates you and then punch a hole in the cup with a pencil or biro. Think of some more things that you have to put up with, and for every one, punch another hole.

If you put your mind to it you can probably come up with at least 30–100 different things. Some of mine would include a stain on my settee that I haven't managed to get off, a button hanging off my coat that needs a quick stitch, a new picture that needs hanging, the spare room which needs tidying before anyone can come and stay, a letter I should have answered by now... and then there's the car, which is well overdue for a wash.

The list is endless, but you get the idea. That paper cup represents your mental energy reserve, so you can imagine with all these holes energy is just draining out of you. Try pouring some water into it – over the sink – and you will see exactly what I mean! With that amount of energy being lost it is no wonder we just don't have the mental stamina to keep going and reach our goals. The cost of ignoring those energy bandits and their draining effect is significant. Even the minor 'one day I will get round to it' jobs deplete your mental resources – they might seem trivial, but their effect on your energy reserves is not.

Opposite are some more examples of 'energy bandits'. Take a moment or two now to jot down as many as you can think of. Then use that list to start to clear them. Try tackling some of the very smallest ones first – those that will only take a minute or two to resolve. Then you will be ready to face some of the others that may be harder and take more work. However many you manage to eliminate, I promise you that the result of blocking those energy leaks will be remarkable. Try it.

COMMON ENERGY LEAKS

■ Unresolved conflicts.

■ Untidy or unclean rooms.

■ Neglected decoration and maintenance of the home.

■ Unclear boundaries. Boundaries are those invisible lines we draw around us to protect us from the consequences of other people's behaviour. For example, if your morning yoga is constantly interrupted by someone, you have a weak boundary. To strengthen it you must ask them to stop disturbing you during your yoga time and if necessary explain the consequences if they fail to respect your request.

■ Clutter that needs sorting.

■ Old clothes that should be given away.

■ Old love letters from past lovers that may need destroying or wrapping in ribbon!

■ Unsupportive friendships. Maybe you need to talk to your friends, or even let them go.

■ Unprocessed mail/paperwork. Remember the 3 Ds – Do it, Delegate it, or Dump it!

■ Procrastination and dithering. For example, you can give yourself and others too much choice when it comes to decision-making. When you are trying to make arrangements it is so much quicker to say 'Friday at 10 or Sunday at 5?', rather than 'When shall I see you?'

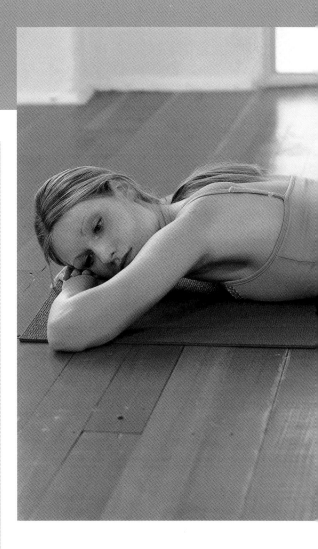

Losing fat and having a joyful life start with a choice and require your attention to maintain. This attention needs both physical and mental energy to fuel it. In this chapter you have started to address this important issue. You probably have never approached weight loss in this way before, but you can see that it makes so much more sense to focus on and make changes to your own inner world than to try to find answers outside yourself. Well done.

The Postures: Part One

Always remember to do your warm-up before you begin (see pages 22–31).

1. Firm Base

1 Stand with your feet at least 1m (3ft) apart, and with your toes turned out at a 45° angle. Bend the knees until you are in a comfortable squat, but ensure that your hips are not lower than your knees.

2 Raise both arms out to the side at shoulder height, turning your palms uppermost.

3 Sweep the arms up to bring your palms together over the top of your head.

4 Bring your arms back down, palms still together, and pause with them in front of your heart. As you do this think of bringing down a higher power (be it God, nature, cosmic consciousness, light, healing, unconditional love, or however else you experience this – use any word or image that works well for you and will help you to achieve slimming success). In this prayer position your hands are forming a *mudra*, which is a symbolic hand gesture used either to seal or circulate energy in specific areas of your body. Hold this position for 30 seconds, breathing normally.

5 Gently come back to standing position by pushing down on to the heels, turning back your toes until they are parallel again, and bringing your feet together. Bring your hands back to your sides and stand like this for a few seconds, noticing how you feel. This final position is the Mountain posture (see page 31).

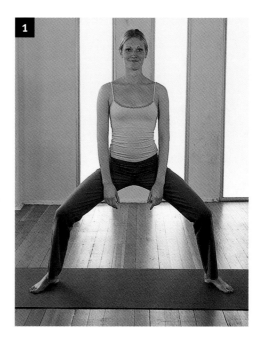

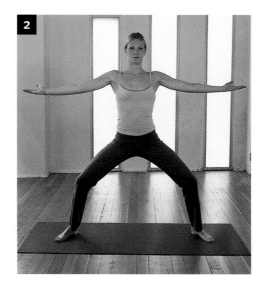

Benefits	
Body	Helps to increase the efficiency of your metabolism by toning the leg muscles (and toned muscles burn calories).
Mind	I can and I will.
Spirit	Anchoring the help you need.

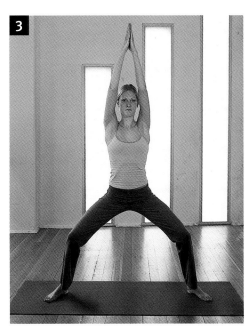

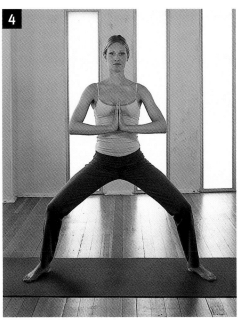

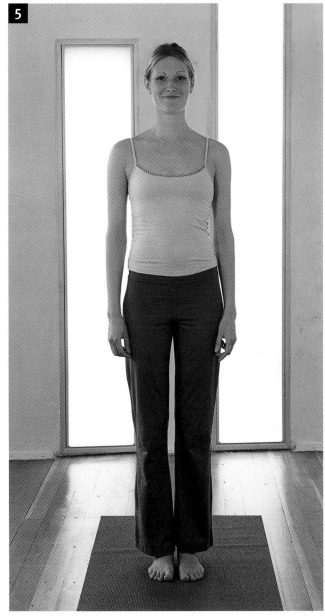

2. Triangle (Trikonasana)

1 Move your feet about 1–1.25m (3–4ft) apart (the distance will vary according to your flexibility and leg length). Turn your left foot out 90° so that it is pointing directly to the left. Point your right foot slightly inwards and line up the instep with your left heal.

2 Inhale and raise your arms out to the side at shoulder height, keeping your palms facing downwards, and look towards your left hand. Feel a strong stretch along your arms to your fingertips and notice your chest expanding. Imagine that your heart is being filled with love.

3 Exhale and reach a little further to the left, then reach down, still maintaining this outstretched feeling without tipping forwards or backwards, as though you were standing between two sheets of glass.

■ Hold on to any part of your leg that you can reach comfortably. You may touch the floor, depending on your flexibility and limb length.

■ Extend your right arm, pointing it directly upwards, and turning the thumb so that it is in line with your shoulder. Gently ease your right

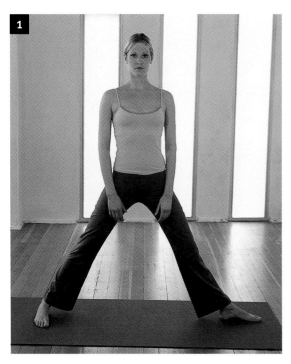

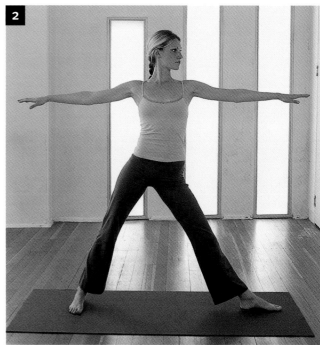

hip back a little. Extend your spine from its base to your neck and maintain an uplifted feeling in the posture. Breathe naturally, dropping any unnecessary tension. Hold for your 4–7 breaths.

4 To come out, inhale; straighten up slowly, stretch your arms out to the side at shoulder height (as in picture 2), then bring your feet together and hands to your sides, so you are in the Mountain posture.

■ Repeat on the other side.

TIP – We need to be strong and put ourselves first if we want to achieve a slimmer, fitter body. The difference between fat and weight loss is that whenever you lose weight it's not necessarily fat – it can be fluid. That is why using scales as an indication of weight loss can be misleading. What we are aiming to do is to lose unnecessary body fat. The ideal fat ratio for a woman should be between 18 per cent and 25 per cent of her total body weight. (Body fat analysers are usually available at your local chemist's.)

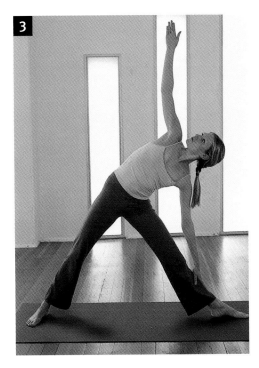

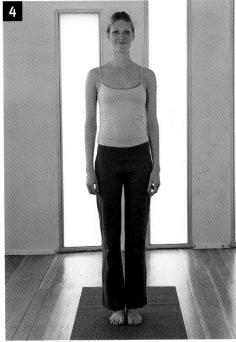

3. Warrior (Virabhadrasana)

1 Stand with your feet approximately 1m (3ft) apart. Turn your left foot out 90° and your right foot in slightly. Align your left heel with your right instep.

■ Breathe in as you raise your arms out to the side at shoulder height, palms facing forwards. Feel your emotional heart opening like a blossoming rose as you stretch along your arms all the way to your fingertips.

2 As you breathe out, gently lunge to the left by bending your left knee (but no more than 90°), and turn your head to look at your left thumb pointing upwards, the fingertips pointing directly away as though indicating your new path – the way to the slim you. The fingers and thumb on the right hand are similarly placed.

■ Feel strong and know you can and WILL succeed. Focus on the thumb nail – learn to spearhead your focus/intention (precision thinking). You are developing the power to make choices.

■ Hold, breathing normally for the recommended 4–7 breaths, and then return to the centre.

■ Repeat on the other side.

TIP – Keep your bent knee above your ankle. If it goes beyond the ankle, ease off and move your legs wider apart.

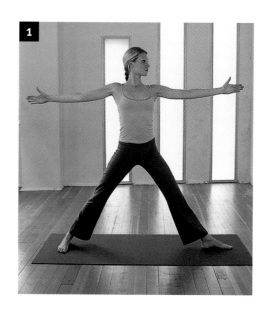

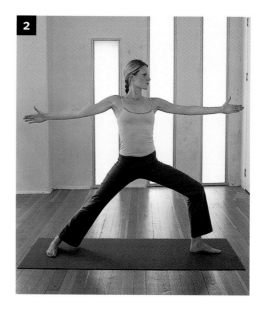

Benefits	
Body	Improves posture and spinal alignment.
Mind	I bring focus to the present.
Spirit	Connectedness.

4. Mountain (Tadasana)

1 Stand with your feet together and hands relaxed by your sides, looking straight ahead. Feel equal weight on each foot and lift yourself 2 or 3cm (1in) taller.

■ Stand in the Mountain pose to bring yourself back to your centre. Feel a sense of joy – and if you don't feel it, then act as if you do.

■ The posture reminds you to release the past that does not serve you and be totally in the present. This is very important when you are held back by feelings of frustration and defeat that come from your history of dieting challenges. A mountain is firm and strong, and so are you.

TIP – Avoid using the word 'problem'. Re-name problems 'opportunities' or 'challenges' – successful people do.

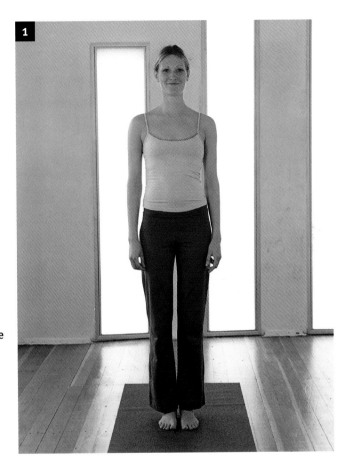

5 Think Big!

I am going to introduce you to a unique and revolutionary concept in slimming: to lose weight, think big. No, I am not crazy. This theory is based on my own experience as well as that of thousands of women who have attended my fitness club, and it took shape when I realised that for so many women, their weight becomes such a fixation that they see everything from the perspective of their size. But for slimming success the real focus should be on the solution rather than the problem – or, as we learned to call it in the last chapter, the challenge! And that solution is that you develop yourself and your capabilities and find your real identity, rather than thinking of yourself as 'fat'. You are much bigger than your size.

Picture perfect

The best way I know to do this is to make up a collage of things in your life that inspire you, or that you really want to happen. It can consist of photos, words, things cut out from magazines or anything that has meaning for you. Put them on a board or in a frame that you can hang on the wall, so that you get to see them regularly every day. The main purpose of the collage is to depict who you are, and perhaps where you have come from and where you aspire to be. When I completed mine it made me feel so proud of the person I was, but at the same time excited by the fact that I still had to realise my full potential! I no longer saw myself as a woman who had struggled with her weight all her life. This was a truly defining 'I'm a swan, not an ugly duckling'

moment. Then, as I discovered that there were some great things I wanted to do in this lifetime, my sense of self and all that I could do opened up before me. Alongside that was the sense of achievement that I derived from remembering the things I'd succeeded at but that had been forgotten when all my attention had just been focused on my being fat. As I did that, I stopped being obsessed by weight (my 'affliction' as I used to call it) and opened myself up to the good things in life. Try it yourself. Create a positive picture image of who you truly are. If you can, please avoid censoring anything that you have chosen, just stick them all up. Remember, your subconscious loves pictures, and you will be delighted with the result. Do it this week!

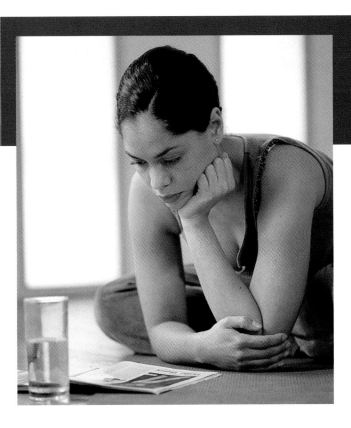

The media

As women, we are no doubt seriously affected by the media image of us that appears every day in magazines, newspapers, on television and in films. It stands to reason that when we fail to live up to the superimposed image of what we 'should' look like, we become discontented with our bodies. Naturally, this discontent spreads, and touches the rest of our lives, including the people around us. Perhaps many of you are not overweight at all, yet still feel discontented because you think you should be 'perfect'. As I've told you before, during all these years working in the health and fitness industry, I've only ever met one woman who was happy with her body. This is bad news indeed, but the good news is that if we can look outward, 'think big' when we come to our self-image and start to expand our creative, loving side, this will be reflected in our bodies. Then that perfect body we all crave (sometimes with disastrous and expensive results) ceases to be the be-all-and-end-all. Life is about so much more than being the ideal weight. If you can accept that, you will lose fat and attract a slimmer body without any of that all-too-familiar striving, fear-based tension and stress. You will get your energy not from the conventional approach ('the uphill struggle will get me there') but from the natural, flowing energy that comes from joyful living. This approach is so much healthier and sustainable, and will result in successful weight management.

Be aware

Awareness allows you to look at things as they are. This is essential, for only when you see things as they are can you change them (if you wish). Awareness is therefore vitally important in our Yoga for Weight Loss programme. Yoga brings both awareness and clarity. We need awareness to see what we truthfully need to change, and indeed can change, but clarity is also about realising what we cannot change; if, like me, you realise that you have a bone structure that makes you look bigger than you are, then you need to think about other ways to help you to look great, like illusion dressing, or using colour and style differently. Let me give you an example.

During most of my 'slimming career' (that is from the age of 16 when I had so-called 'puppy fat'), I had been pursuing the ideal body. Sadly it wasn't my body I was searching for, so bar a miracle happening to make my bone structure elongate around the middle I was stuck. However... miracles do happen, and I had a change of awareness. I had always judged myself by how I look in a bikini – most women do. The miracle happened when I finally realised that my body is very short-waisted and does not look good in a bikini, full stop. I can be slim as a pin, but wearing a bikini is never going to flatter me – it just isn't me! You have no idea how much pain and despair this caused me at first. But it led me to the discovery of how colour can either enhance or detract from your looks. I discovered that a bright pink bikini was not appropriate or suitable for me, but put me in a chocolate-brown swimming costume and I looked great. And for all those years I thought the problem was solely my weight.

We also need awareness to be focused on what we are eating. That's why slimming clubs encourage you to write down everything you eat, which is a very helpful practice. It is all too easy to eat without really being aware of eating. In my own case I remember frequently thinking that my husband had eaten all the cheese in the fridge. Eventually I complained to him about it, and when he said he hadn't eaten any at all, I had a rude awakening. I realised it was me who kept going to the fridge and pinching bits of cheese. Subconsciously I knew I was doing it, but I was kidding myself I wasn't, because I was not aware. Have you ever had the experience of catching sight of all the empty wine bottles on the table after a dinner party, but having no recollection at all of everyone getting through so many? You simply didn't notice how much was being drunk. Awareness brings acceptance, and acceptance of yourself, right now, will bring empowerment.

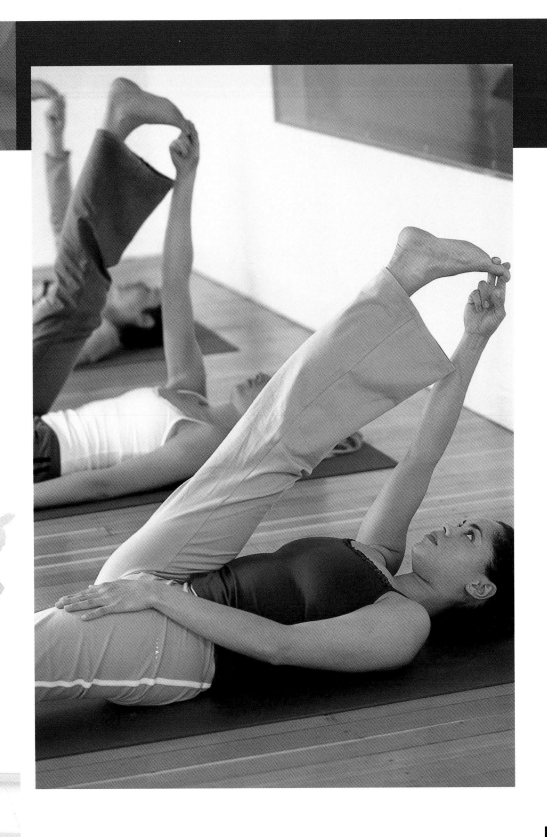

Benefits	
Body	Fires up the digestion and tones the abdominal muscles.
Mind	I am in control.
Spirit	Power.

5. Yogic Tummy Tuck (Uddiyana Bandha)

This is a good pose to do in a weight management programme because it can fire up the digestion. However, treat this one with caution, and don't do it if you have an IUD fitted, have any internal abdominal illness, or have had or need any operations in that area. Miss this one out also if you are having your period. Your stomach and bowels should be fairly empty before attempting this.

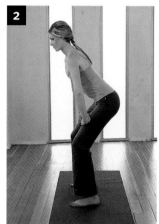 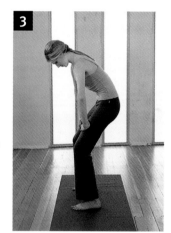 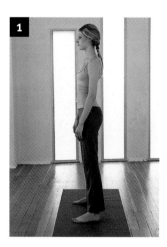

1 Stand upright with your feet about 60cm (2ft) apart, toes slightly turned out.

2 Take a deep breath in, bend the knees a little and allow the back to soften and be rounded. Place both hands on your thighs, fingertips pointing inwards, and support the weight of your torso on your arms.

■ Exhale completely, expelling all the air from your lungs and abdominal area through the mouth.

3 Now draw the abdomen inwards and upwards, creating a deep hollow.

■ Flap the tummy in and out in a wave-like motion 10–20 times and then, when you need to inhale, do so, and stand upright again. After a few normal breaths you are ready to repeat.

■ Repeat the exercise twice more if you wish.

Benefits	
Body	Stretches the back of the body and stimulates the brain.
Mind	I see things as they are.
Spirit	At one with nature.

6. Inverted 'V' (Adhomukha Svanasana)

1 Stand with your feet parallel, about 60cm (2ft) apart, with knees soft.

2 Walk both hands down your body and on to the ground, and continue walking them out until your body is bent at the hips, forming a right-angle. Your hands are just wider than shoulder-width apart, the middle fingers pointing directly forward.

■ Try to extend the length of your spine by keeping the buttocks high. Hold this position for your 4–7 breaths.

3 To come out, bend the knees towards the ground and go on to all fours with your toes down flat, ready for the next posture.

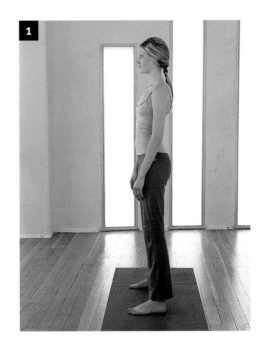

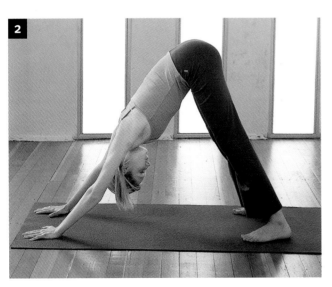

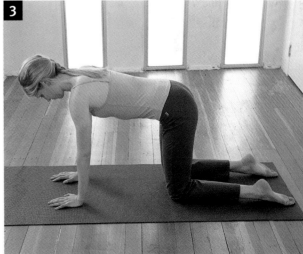

7. Contract, Expand, Balance

Balance is so important in a weight-loss programme. If you deprive yourself too much your body will want to redress the balance, and it's hardly surprising that you will then go and grab a chocolate bar. According to the ancient yogic scriptures we need to have balance in our lives – do not overeat, do not undereat – and this requires a good, healthy, common-sense approach to exercise and dieting.

I love the teachings of the balance postures. If we lived our lives in accordance with nature and our feelings, there are times when we would need to withdraw and regenerate. Sadly, our unnatural lives dictate that we have to overwork, and we do not have the luxury of withdrawing when our bodies tell us to – when we are ill, or when we feel the need to get away, whether this is to an actual retreat or just somewhere quiet to 'top up the batteries'. It is said that, in ancient times, on the full moon or when they were menstruating, women would be honoured by their communities for their intuitive wisdom. It was expected (and necessary) that the women would withdraw from community life. They would chant together or spend time in reflection in a loving group. Nowadays we have our period and we just have to get on with it. By using the symbolism of this posture we can help to

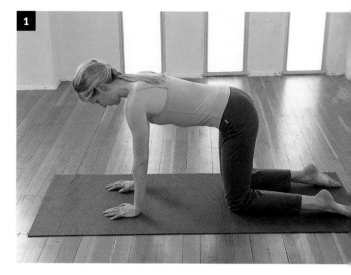

honour that need to contract and expand, and thus bring balance back into our lives. Balancing postures also naturally help to calm the mind. Try doing this in an agitated state and you will find it harder to balance.

1 Lean on all fours, with your hands aligned beneath your shoulders and knees underneath the hips. Keep your spine and neck in a straight line, so that you are looking at the floor.

2 As you exhale, gently bring your left knee in towards your forehead, hold.

3 Extend your right arm and left leg out as you breathe in and hold the balance. Your right arm and left leg will be parallel to the ground, outstretched. Hold for your 4–7 breaths and come back to the all-fours position.

■ Repeat on the other side.

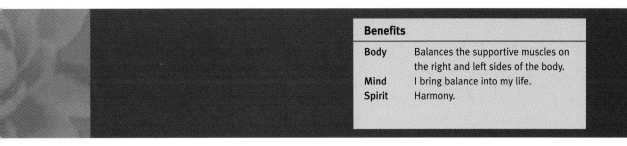

Benefits

Body	Balances the supportive muscles on the right and left sides of the body.
Mind	I bring balance into my life.
Spirit	Harmony.

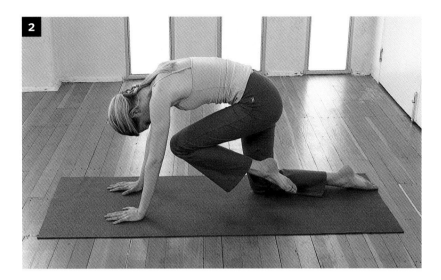

TIP – To help you balance, practise with just the leg only to start with and then bring the arm up when you are feeling more confident.

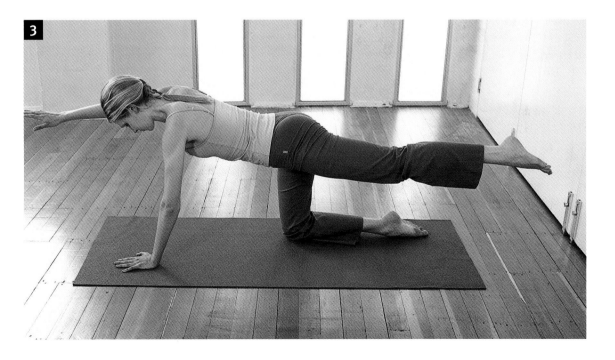

8. Plank (Chaturanga Dandasana)

Easier option –

1 Start in your all-fours position.

2 Walk your hands, which are placed slightly wider than shoulder-width apart, a few centimetres forward, shifting your shoulder-weight over your wrists, and hold, keeping your back flat. Hold for just a few seconds.

■ Return to the all-fours position.

3 Lower yourself down gently and lie flat on your tummy, putting your hands one on top of the other and resting one cheek on your hands. Take a couple of deep breaths and bring yourself back to your centre.

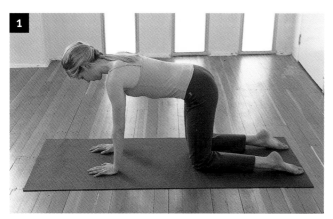

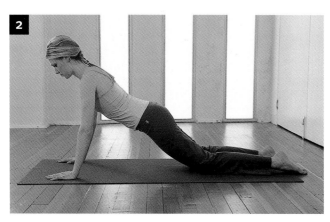

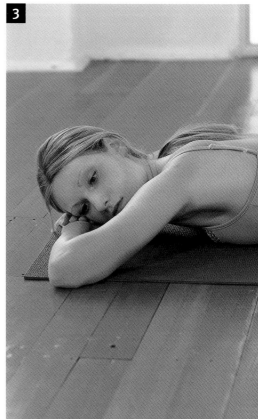

Benefits	
Body	Helps tone the muscles that support the breasts and therefore helps prevent sagging, and tones the abdominal muscles.
Mind	I can and I will.
Spirit	Strength.

Advanced version –

4 Follow stages 1 and 2 (see opposite), then curl your toes under and straighten the body from your head to your toes, feet hip-distance apart, hands just wider than shoulder-width, arms straight but not locked. The body should be flat like a plank. Hold for your 4–7 breaths.

■ Lower yourself down gently and lie flat on your tummy, putting your hands one on top of the other and resting one cheek on your hands. Take a couple of deep breaths and bring yourself back to your centre (see picture 3, opposite).

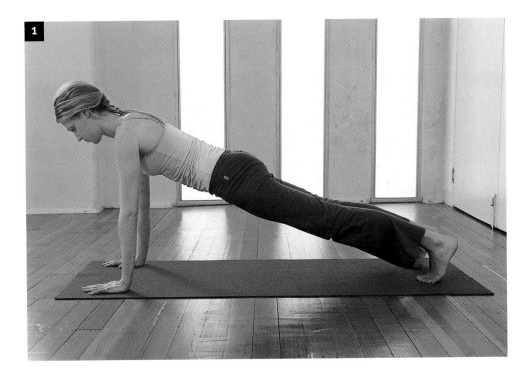

TIP – Allow yourself to do the easier version to begin with; it is much better to do that than to overexert yourself and regret it later.

6 Learning to Love and Forgive

In the last chapter we talked about changing the vision you have of yourself and thinking bigger in order to appreciate yourself. Now we are going to go a little deeper. I want you to look at how you truly feel about yourself and how willing you are to love yourself unconditionally, whatever your present shape. I know it is not always easy when you have spent a lot of time criticising and judging. I used to have a sticker on the scales at my fitness club that said, 'I love myself,' and I am sure that most people thought it was weird. However, nowadays the importance of these personal messages we give ourselves is generally accepted, and self-understanding has become recognised as a powerful key to making fundamental changes in our lives. It is time we truly become aware of the fact that we need to love ourselves exactly as we are, right now. And remember, it is said that unless we love ourselves, we cannot truly love others.

In the past I would treat myself so badly, bingeing on food and alcohol, and staying in a boring job because I didn't feel I was good enough for anything else. And it took me quite a while to realise that I needed to treat myself as my own best friend, because that is who I am. What kind of a best friend is always criticising you? Our friends love us despite our faults, so I am going to ask you to love yourself exactly like that. It doesn't matter if you are twice the size you want to be, or even if you have lots more fat than you would wish for – you can love yourself right now, just as you are, without changing anything except your own attitude. If you find it difficult to love yourself,

try standing in front of a mirror and saying 'I love you' to yourself at least a hundred times every day. I did this many years ago, thinking it was absolutely stupid, but I kept with it, and it worked! So do try it.

Forgiveness is very important, both for you and for others. I believe that negative emotions 'congest' the body and anything that psychologically congests also causes physical congestion. Remember that the mind and body are linked, and if you are holding on to negative emotions that congestion might manifest itself in your body as you holding on to extra weight or finding it hard to release fat. That is because congestion causes – you've

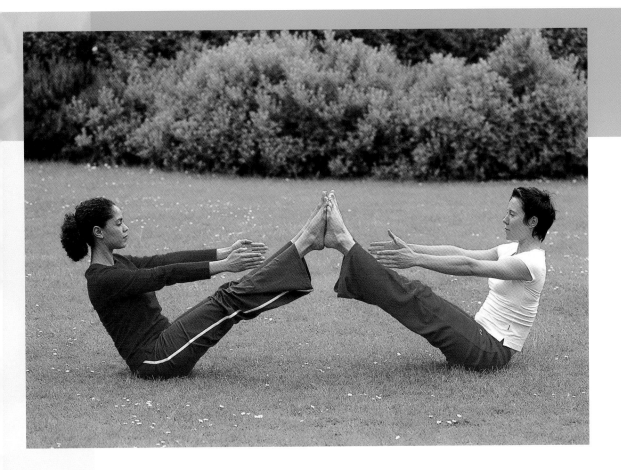

guessed it – fat or water retention, and prevents the body working efficiently, thus causing more congestion and establishing a negative cycle. Now we definitely do NOT want anything like that to happen if we have weight challenges, because we want to make things as simple as possible for ourselves.

A clearer way ahead

It is important to remember that our mind rarely perceives things as they truly are. It operates largely from a state of false understanding, often supplying us with inaccurate data. If a false premise we have about ourselves remains unchallenged it becomes our truth. For instance, when you look in a mirror are you really seeing yourself as you are, or through the judgements and opinions of others about how you 'ought' to look? Women in particular suffer from this false image of themselves and when we base our actions on such inaccurate information, we inadvertently create a great deal of unnecessary suffering. It is crucial that we maintain clarity of perception – this can determine the success of our slimming endeavours and weight control afterwards. Practising forgiveness in our lives, towards ourselves and others, can substantially help to clean the window through which we see ourselves and the world that surrounds us.

Forgiveness is one of the most self-empowering actions I know, and anything that helps us to feel empowered is absolutely vital in our choice to be slim.

So okay, you say, there is forgiveness and forgiveness. If you have lived a fairly normal life (whatever that is!), you will probably have your own personal bank of forgiveness issues which hold varying degrees of 'charge', especially around weight issues. Let's look at some examples. Can you forgive and forget:

- The children at school who taunted you and called you 'Fattie'?
- Parents who told you to eat up all our food, even when you were full?
- Relatives who rewarded you with cakes and sweets?
- Strangers who made rude comments about your size?
- The media who portray a long thin body as an ideal?
- Those people who can eat what they want and not put an ounce of fat on?
- Occasions when there is pressure to eat lots of highly fattening food?

These are the ones that are particularly relevant for me, but I am sure you can think of more that mean something to you. Be honest and bring to mind all those people or circumstances that you blame.

Sit down somewhere quiet where you will not be disturbed and just let yourself forgive them. Thinking of them and saying 'I forgive you' out loud or quietly to yourself will be fine. Sometimes this brings up strong emotions and you may need a box of tissues handy as a healthy emotional release may occur.

However, if you have very deep emotional issues relating to trauma or abuse in your past, then you may need professional help. Using a book about forgiveness may also be helpful, and it may be enough initially for you to have just the wish to forgive. When I had such a problem, I found that asking a higher power to help me to forgive eased my feelings immensely. You do not have to see that person again – just forgiving them in your mind will help you greatly.

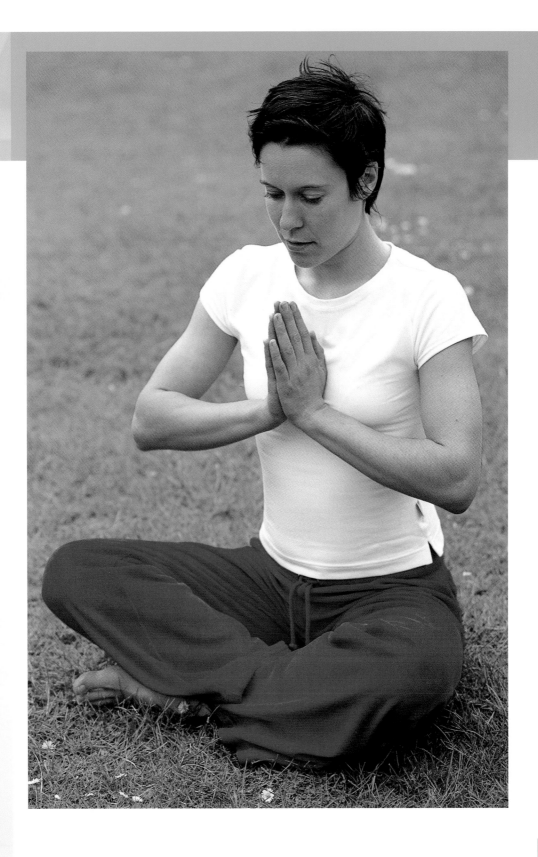

The Postures: Part Three

Benefits

Body	Stretches the chest, tones the upper body and rejuvenates the spine.
Mind	I look forward to being the new, slim me.
Spirit	Transformation.

9. Transformation (Bhujanasana)

Back bends bring exhilaration and a sense of moving forwards. During our daily lives most of our movements involve bending forwards and activities in front of the body – for example, working at a desk, holding a baby, writing, doing housework, preparing and cooking food – so back bends re-balance our whole system.

1 Lie face down on your abdomen, and pause. Place your hands on the ground with your fingertips pointing forwards level with your shoulders. (If you are new to this posture take your hands 30cm [1ft] in front of your shoulders and over the coming weeks bring them closer to the shoulders.) Keep your feet together and tense your buttocks slightly.

2 Breathe in and raise your head and shoulders without using your arms at first. This will help develop strength in your back. Then use your arms to bring yourself up to a position where you feel a curve in your spine, but with your hips on the ground. Elbows are soft (that is, not locked straight).

■ Hold for 7 breaths, or less if you are new to this. Keep your shoulders relaxed, elbows close in to the body and chin parallel to the ground. Do it twice, holding for 2 breaths if this is easier for you.

■ Breathe normally. Acknowledge your willingness to transform and change. Change is always frightening, and although achieving the shape you desire seems a blissful notion, it can be scary at some level. Affirm your willingness to move beyond this and accept all the responsibility and consequences that a new slimmer you will bring.

■ Slowly lower your body and relax.

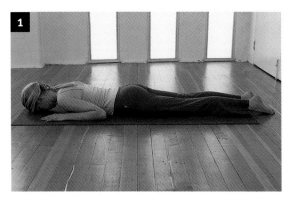

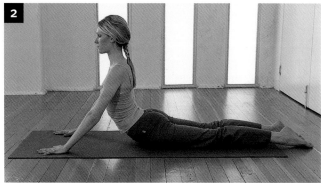

Benefits	
Body	Releases tension in the shoulders and hips.
Mind	I am perfect as I am.
Spirit	Unconditional love.

10. Child Pose (Balasana)

1 Kneel down, sitting back on your heels, with your toes flat on the floor.

2 Slowly bend forwards, allowing your forehead to rest on the ground. Use a cushion under your forehead if it's more comfortable.

■ Relax your arms by your sides and the backs of your hands on the ground. Your buttocks should be kept towards your heels and your toes should be flat on the ground.

■ Become aware of your breath. As you breathe in your tummy expands and as you breathe out it contracts. Hold for your 4–7 breaths.

3 To come out of this pose, lift yourself up slowly, uncurl your body and finally raise your shoulders and head.

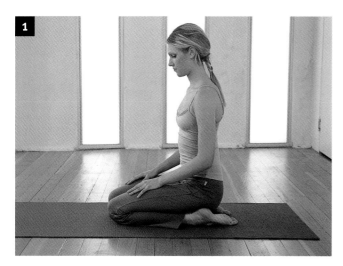

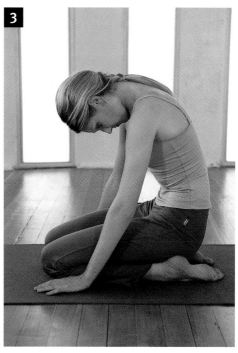

11. Hug Yourself

When was the last time you received a hug, or gave a hug? It makes you feel good, doesn't it? Our body loves being given hugs, especially by itself. Well, you are going to give yourself a great big hug, right now.

1 Lie flat on your back with your knees bent and feet flat on the floor, hip-distance apart.

2 Wrap your arms around you so that you are holding your shoulders; your elbows should be pointing up towards the ceiling

3 Hold for a few moments, then pull in your tummy muscles and, keeping your feet still and legs and pelvis stationary, rock your elbows from side to side. Keep looking at the ceiling, and feel your upper back being massaged and your spine getting a healing rock. Do this 7 times on to each side.

■ Lie flat in Rejuvenation Posture (see pages 24–5) for 2 breaths, bringing yourself back to a place of being totally in the here and now.

TIP – Appreciate yourself, love yourself, and value yourself – if you don't you won't be able to allow anyone else to.

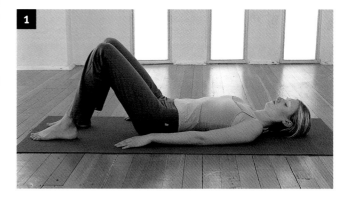

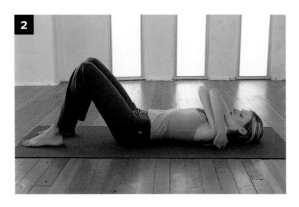

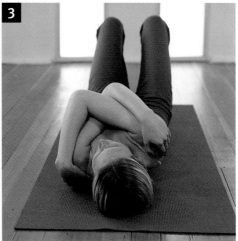

Benefits	
Body	Increases flexibility in the spine and optimises the working of the thyroid gland.
Mind	I am open to new ways of thinking.
Spirit	Support.

12. Bridge (Uttana Mayurasana)

1 Lie flat on the floor, with your feet flat on the ground hip-distance apart, bringing your heels towards your buttocks.

2 Keeping your arms on the floor, palms down, slowly raise your buttocks off the floor. Hold in the uppermost position, arching your spine and lifting your hips up towards the ceiling as far as is comfortable.

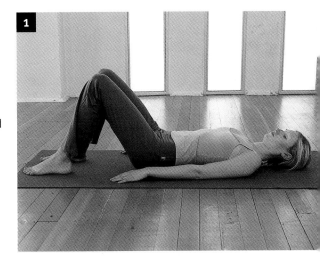

3 Feel the rise and fall of the abdominal muscles as you breathe in and out. When you are ready, lower the spine, upper back first, and finally push your buttocks towards your heels.

■ Extend the legs out straight and lie still for a few seconds.

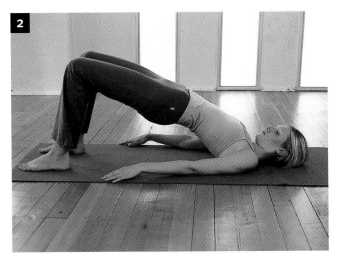

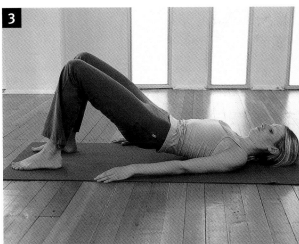

7 Believe in Yourself

In the previous chapters, we examined at the truth about who we are and how we look. This glimpse of who we truly are does in itself help us to feel in control because we no longer see through 'fat-tinted' spectacles. I have a great example of this. Before I managed to change my perception in this way, when my period was due I honestly felt that I had put on about 2 stone (13kg) overnight. Somehow in my deluded mind I really believed it, until one day I asked my husband, Pete: 'Have I put on 2 stone since yesterday?' Of course, his answer was a straightforward 'No!' I may have been suffering from water retention, but there was no way I had put on 2 stone overnight! So a good question to ask yourself is 'Is this really true?'

Being in control means seeing things as they are, and turning your back on false thinking and the sense of panic you feel when you seem to have lost your grip on things. If you stick with the Yoga for Weight Loss programme you will start to feel in control. Just practise the yoga sequence each day, with faith, love and determination, for one month. It's about making a commitment to yourself, so you cannot afford to make exceptions: take time off only if you are ill or it's absolutely impossible for you to fit it into your day.

Limiting beliefs

Most people have powerful beliefs about themselves and about 'what's right', especially when it comes to food and slimming. Unfortunately many of these beliefs are subconscious thoughts that you are unaware of, so you cannot challenge them.

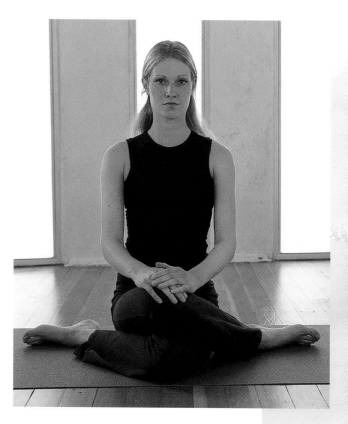

Many of the thoughts that you have are conditionings or default thoughts and are never questioned – they just come up automatically and you may not even register them. If you do not challenge them, however, they become your truth. In the past you may have tried to slim and not succeeded, but is the statement 'I can't slim' really true? These limiting beliefs form your patterns of behaviour. For example, if you believe that food gives you comfort, you will comfort eat. Try now to think of three limiting beliefs that you have. If you need some reassurance that you are not alone, here are some beliefs that my students and I have shared:

■ I can't go out for a meal without putting on weight.
■ I always put on weight on holidays.
■ I only have to look at a biscuit to put on weight.
■ Just one small drink won't matter.
■ I have to finish the whole packet otherwise they will go off.
■ Losing weight is always hard and I always fail, so what is the point?

Write your own limiting beliefs – three at least – on a scrap of paper, then have a little ceremony to challenge them and get rid of them. The mind loves rituals. Rituals draw

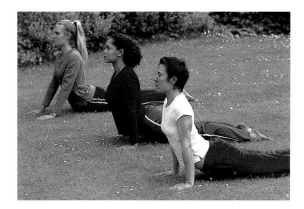

attention to what you are doing and what your intention is, so scrunch your piece of paper up and burn it, flush it down the loo or tear it into tiny pieces. Say out loud that these limiting beliefs will no longer hold you back in your quest for a life free from weight challenges.

Fear

Fear of being fat and of getting fatter holds us back from being slim. Admitting and understanding you are fearful will help. We don't like to admit to being fearful, but owning up to it is very empowering. I found that the more I was fearful of putting on weight, the more I seemed to do so. This in itself was very stressful, and I overate as a consequence. Watch out for fear and how it makes you eat. Avoid fearful situations as much as possible – this could be anything from weighing yourself too often or not having the courage to say no

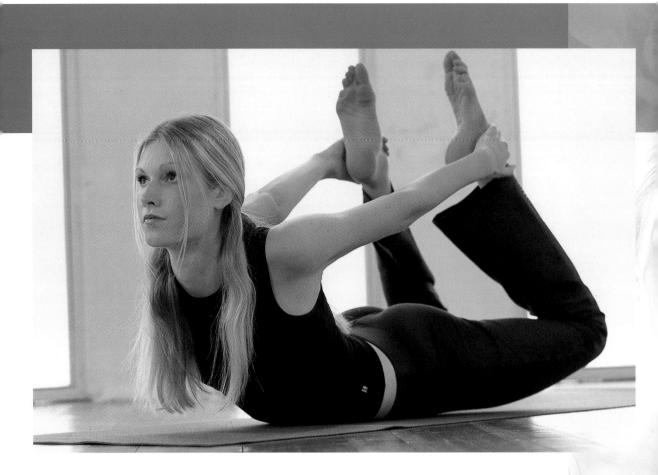

to fattening food on social occasions, to being pushed too far too soon at work; even a joy ride at the fair could trigger adrenalin and set you off eating. Yoga for Weight Loss will help to make you stronger, in body, mind and spirit, so fear will not be such a challenge.

Will-power

I have heard too many women say 'I've no will-power'. They bring up their children, hold down a demanding job, keep a relationship and home together, but just because they fall down when it comes to keeping a slim figure they say they have no strength of will. If this is something that you recognise in yourself, then please let's change it to 'I find keeping slim challenging, but I'll get there!' Let's not delude ourselves here: losing weight and sticking to a health programme are hard challenges because we are bombarded with adverts of slim people stuffing food down on television and in magazines and yet they never put on weight! To say nothing of the temptation that awaits us in every shop and supermarket checkout area where there is always a huge display of crisps, sweets and chocolates facing you. Let's redress the balance. Think of all the other areas of your life where you do have immense will-power. Think of at least two, and then write them down.

■ When I support someone, I always get them to write down their accomplishments in life before we get started, from learning to drive to getting a promotion or being involved in a sport or hobby. Take a good look back at your life so far and then write down at least five things you have done that that you are pleased, or proud of, and you will notice that you actually did exert plenty of will-power to achieve them.

....
....
....
....
....
....
....
....
....
....
....
....
....
....

The Postures:
Part Four

Benefits

Body	Makes the spine more flexible.
Mind	I annihilate negative thinking.
Spirit	Bliss.

13. Knees-together Twist (Supta Parivartanasana I)

This posture will help you develop strong self-belief.

1 Lie on your back. Bring both knees, pressed together, up to your chest.

■ Take your arms out to the side and lay them flat on the floor, palms down, at shoulder level.

2 Slowly lower your knees to one side as far as is comfortable, keeping your shoulders on the floor and knees together. Face the opposite direction to your knees. Hold for your 4–7 breaths.

■ Repeat on the other side, then come back to the centre and lower the legs to the floor.

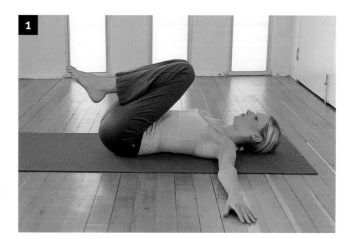

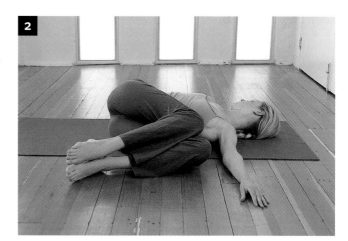

Benefits

Body	Helps to detoxify the body.
Mind	I see things clearly.
Spirit	Purification.

14. Cleanse and Twist
(Supta Parivartanasana II)

I love this posture, and if I could take only one yoga
posture to a desert island this is the one I would choose.

1 Lie flat on the floor, checking that your body is symmetrical.

■ Relax your head.

■ Place your right foot on top of your left knee and twist your knee to the left. Keep both shoulders flat on the floor. The left hand can be placed gently on the right thigh, but take care not to apply too much pressure.

■ Take the right hand out in line with your shoulder, palm uppermost, and look towards it.

■ Hold for approximately 7 breaths.

■ Return to the centre, relax flat on the floor and again check the symmetry of your body.

■ Repeat on the other side.

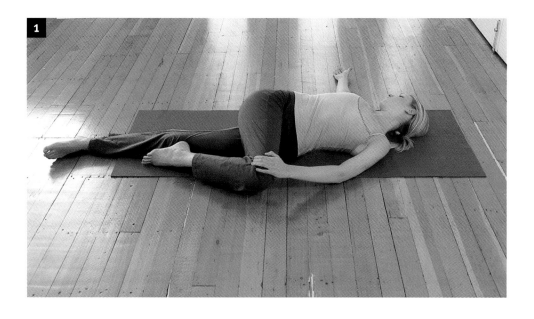

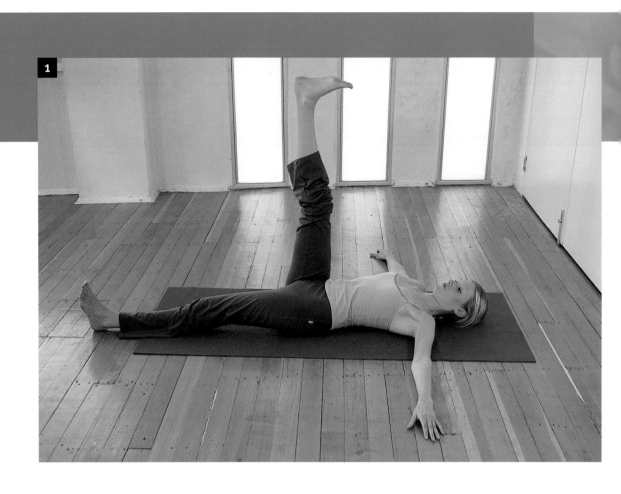

15. Leg Raise into Maltese Cross (Supta Padangusthasana)

In this posture allow your mind to do the work; give it control. Let your mind move your legs – let it be a conscious act.

1 Lie on your back with your legs stretched out and arms out to the side at shoulder level, palms flat on the floor. Lift your straightened right leg to a vertical position, or as far as you can lift it comfortably with your lower back flat on the floor. You can make this more of a challenge by pushing your heel away.

■ Keep your back flat on the floor, stay focused and practise controlling your mind, stopping it from wandering. Bringing conscious control to postures will train your flabby 'choice muscles' to select the right food for your body and the right-sized portions without effort. The mind can help us most when it is fully conscious.

Benefits

Body	Tones and balances the muscles of the lower body.
Mind	My mind is made up and strong.
Spirit	Radiance.

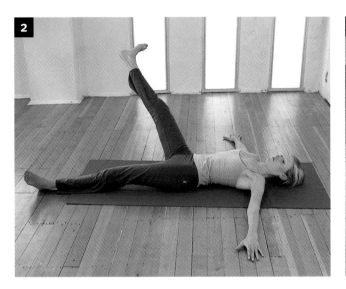

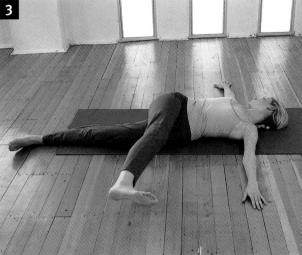

2 Keeping your straightened leg high, gently lower it to your right side, down to the floor as far as it is comfortable. Make sure your left buttock is flat on the floor and does not rise up, so that the hips are parallel to the floor. Keep your foot flexed if you want a harder posture.

3 Hold, and then on inhalation bring the leg back to the vertical position and move it gently across the body to the left side; hold. Again, keep the foot flexed if you want a harder

posture. Keep your head in the centre, looking forward, or turn to face the opposite hand, away from the leg.

■ Breathe in, raise the leg back to the vertical and slowly lower it down alongside the resting leg, keeping the foot flexed. Repeat with the left leg.

TIP – Always remember that the mind can be your greatest enemy or your greatest friend.

Positive Communication

Everything we think or say has an impact on our behaviour, either consciously or unconsciously. You will have heard 'You are what you eat' repeated frequently in articles on health and well-being; well, what if we were to extend the principle to 'I am what I say'? If it were true, what impact do you think it would have? Let's see how it fits in with our new positive self-image.

Power talk

Positive communication, or 'power talk' as I like to call it, inspires us, keeps us positive and on track. What you are probably more familiar with is its exact opposite – negative talk that we use to sabotage ourselves, mostly unwittingly. I am asking you to think about what comes out of your mouth (rather than what goes into it, which is the main thrust of most other slimming programmes). I first noticed and then became interested in power talking when I was greeting people arriving at my health club. Often the first thing they would say as they came through the doors was, 'Morning. Miserable day.' Of course, they were referring to the weather, but subconsciously it had a depressing effect. I got fed up with this and decided to change it around, so I would say in response, 'Yes, it is raining, but it's a wonderful day.' After a few puzzled looks and double-takes they would laugh because they could see how negative they sounded. I constantly challenge negative language, and nowadays, in fact, very little that is not positive or factual comes out of my mouth. The only exception, of course, is when it's true, and then it's acceptable. Another bugbear of mine is the most frequent greeting we give to both friends and acquaintances, that old standby, 'How are you?', to which comes the usual response, 'Okay.' No wonder we just feel mediocre! 'Okay' is not very positive, is it? The next time someone asks you this question, why not try saying, 'I'm bordering on the fantastic!' and see how alive you and they feel. It will certainly jolt the pattern of your conversation and give them pause to wonder what you have been up to!

We all have favourite phrases that we don't even realise we are using, let alone how often we use them. In order to eliminate some of the most negative ones, I have made a list of definite slimmer's 'nos' which I suggest you remove from your vocabulary now and forever. A good question to ask yourself with each of these statements would be: 'Is this really true?'

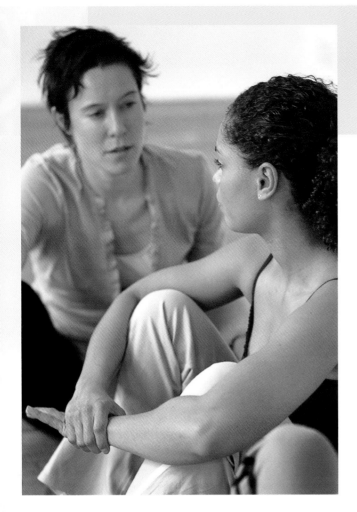

you could devise. If you believe you are no good at it, then of course you are right.

■ 'Every diet I try fails' – a guaranteed outcome if you keep saying that.

■ 'I'm going on holiday so I'm bound to put on a few extra pounds' – again, guaranteed now.

■ 'I've been bad' – usually meaning you have overeaten – and you are looking for a way to punish yourself. This is sad because you are not bad; you are a great person who just at the minute is struggling and has overeaten because you have gone off course.

■ 'I'm shattered.' How exactly? Can you see how, if you really get a handle on your feelings, you could say something like 'I've worked well and I'm really tired, but I'm not prepared to put myself through that level of work and stress again.' You'll be more aware of the state you are in, and less tempted to reach for a sugary snack to boost your depleted energy levels.

■ 'I'm starving' – remember your body is always listening to you, and if you keep saying this it will believe you and help you out by overeating to compensate.

■ 'I'll die if I don't eat something soon' – a very powerful message to eat immediately, and probably anything in sight. Definitely the wrong message!

■ 'I'd give anything for a chocolate' – really? Think of something dear to your heart. Would you swap it for that chocolate?

■ 'I'm no good at dieting' – this is the most powerful way to set yourself up to fail that

You may recognise all of these, but still have a few more that are personal to you. Make a note of them right now and turn them into positives. It might feel and sound false to begin with, but it will become second nature to you – and those around you. You will feel happier and more optimistic and will emerge triumphant from Yoga for Weight Loss programme, which will then, like a pebble thrown into water, send ripples out into the rest of your life.

The Postures: Part Five

16. Shoulder Stand (Sarvangasana)

Do not do this posture if you are pregnant or menstruating, or suffer from heart disease, hypothyroidism, high blood pressure or eye and ear problems that could be aggravated by extra pressure. If you are new to this posture, place a folded blanket under your shoulders (but not your head) so that there is no strain on the neck. If you find this posture in any way difficult, just lie with your feet up on a wall, or on a chair.

Time for a reality check, because in this posture you can get a good look at your tummy hanging down. You may think that this is bad news, but NO, it isn't. It will be very good news when you see less of it – which you surely will when you have completed the programme. This position has often been referred to as 'the mother of postures', because just as a mother brings health and harmony to the home, so this posture brings health and harmony to the whole body.

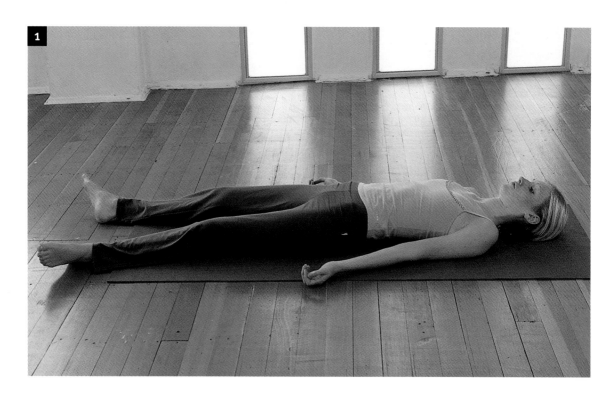

1

Benefits

Body	Works the whole body.
Mind	I accept myself and others from all angles.
Spirit	Truth and perception.

1 Lie on your back with your legs straight and your arms resting alongside your body.

2 Turn the hands over so that your palms are flat on the floor, then, using your arms and hands for support, bend your knees and slowly raise the buttocks, hips and body off the floor.

3 Cup the hips with both hands and support yourself by resting the elbows and upper arms on the floor. Straighten your legs.

■ The body rests comfortably on the shoulders, the nape of the neck and the upper arms. Relax into this position, allowing positivity to flow to body and mind. The chin is well tucked into the chest; this is important as it helps to regulate and optimise the thyroid gland, which is essential to help you control your weight.

■ Focus on bringing your chest to your chin rather than your chin to your chest.

■ Come down by bending the knees and putting your hands back to the floor, palms down, to support the body so that you can lower it slowly down.

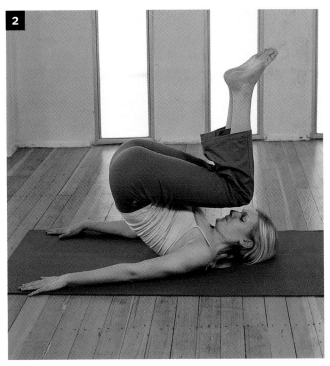

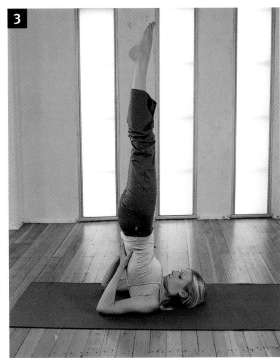

17. Neck Exercise (Brahma Mudra)

If I could encourage you to do just one exercise that will keep you slim for the rest of your life, it would be to practise turning your head from side to side and saying 'No'. Especially when faced with unnecessary or unhealthy food choices. Let's practise this with an important classical yoga posture.

1 Sit in a cross-legged position, with a straight spine. Place your hands gently on your knees or cup them in your lap.

2 Inhale and as you exhale turn your head to the left; when you are ready, inhale and come back to centre.

■ Repeat on the right side. Do this three times each side, and as you do it see yourself in a situation where you want to say no, but seem so far to have lacked the strength of will and accepted that extra glass of wine or piece of cake.

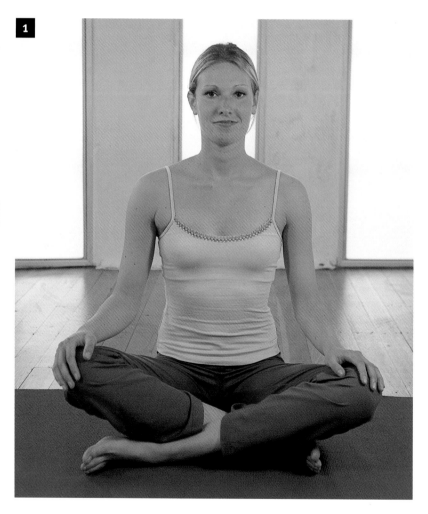

Benefits

Body	Eases tension in the neck muscles and helps tone those dormant 'no' muscles (choice muscles).
Mind	It's okay to say 'No'.
Spirit	Discernment.

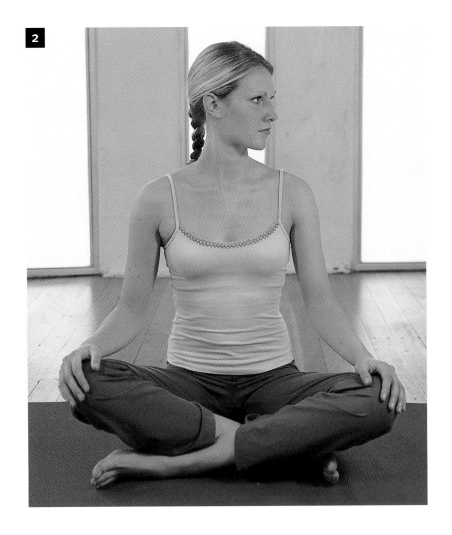

2

9 Feeling Fulfilled

Identifying your personal core values and living by them is an important area of your personal development. A value is something you are naturally drawn to, and eager to do or adopt without effort. If you live according to your values you will feel fulfilled and in harmony with life. People are more often aware of their values when they are young, but as they grow older they 'forget' them. Returning to your values and acting accordingly are important for feeling fulfilled – and successful slimming. This is because a life oriented around your values will be so much enhanced that you will no longer need to reach for food to satisfy yourself – you will feel fulfilled (literally, filled full) in healthier ways.

CORE VALUES

Adventure	Improve	Feel good	Be amused	Kindness
Risk	Facilitate	Be with	Sports	Unconditional
Dare	Provide	In touch	Relate	love
Seek	Help	Lead	Connected	Teach
Experiment	Create	Guide	Family	Educate
Beauty	Design	Influence	Community	Instruct
Attractiveness	Invent	Rule	Nurture	Inform
Loveliness	Imagine	Persuade	Sensitive	Uplift
Magnificence	Plan	Encourage	Tenderness	Explain
Catalyse	Build	Expert	Support	Win
Impact	Inspire	Outdo	Compassion	Accomplish
Encourage	Discover	Excellence	Respond	Triumph
Influence	Learn	Set standards	Spiritual	Attract
Stimulate	Realise	Pleasure	Be aware	
Energise	Discern	Have fun	Be accepting	
Contribute	Observe	Sex	Devotion	
Serve	Feel	Sensual	Enlightenment	

The list opposite contains some of the words that might reflect your values. Circle in pencil at least ten that seem appropriate. Think about them for a few days, see how they 'fit' you, then put them in order of importance from 1 to 10. Use them to help you.

Let's see how this works in practice. We can use me as an example. My own personal values are 'Feel good', 'Loveliness', 'Inspire' and 'Sensual'. Now, with a list like that, a job on an oil rig is obviously not for me. I like to feel good, so I definitely need to put in time and effort to exercise on a regular basis. Eating correctly is also very important to me because if I do eat the wrong things I hate it – I whinge and complain. I have always liked lovely things, preferably fluffy or soft (sensual) things, and I like to inspire by writing books, leading seminars and giving talks. This is part of the package that is the true me. I know not to try to fit myself into the wrong hole, and this saves me time and money and helps me to plan a successful and joyous life. Before I undertake any project, I see if it fits in with my core values. If it doesn't, then I won't waste my time doing it; if I am not acting in accordance with my basic values I cannot live with integrity.

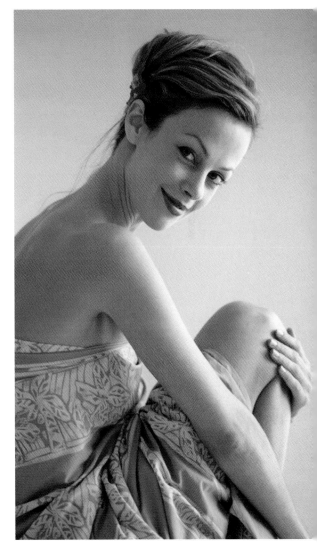

Bear in mind that I use the word 'value' to mean much more than the conventional media definition. We are talking about your values, not the values that society thinks you should hold. At the core of every human being there is uniqueness and individuality that demand to be expressed. There are no exceptions to this rule; it absolutely and definitely includes you. Living according to your personal values, setting your goals or in fact doing anything with reference to your values, enables you to be your unique self. Your goal of slimming will be effortless because your values will draw you; it will not be effortless if you have to push yourself. Fear-based systems such as crash dieting, extreme exercise routines and endless self-sacrifice will all produce tension, and even if you painstakingly reach your slimming goals the tension will catapult you back to being overweight.

To help you visualise this, imagine that someone has wrapped a thick rubber band around your waist and that for each unit of weight you lose you move away from the person holding the other end of the band. Notice the strain of the band resisting against you as move towards your goal weight. This resistance gets harder and harder, and even if you do struggle and reach your goal the tension is still there and inevitably pulls you back to your original weight or worse. This illustrates the common phenomenon known as 'yo-yo dieting'. The Yoga for Weight Loss programme eliminates this tension and instead promotes an effortless way of losing fat and staying slim (what we call 'ho-ho dieting'!).

Setting value-based goals

Now, just for a minute, let's go back and look at the ten values that you circled in the list. Study them hard and in your own time narrow them down to between four and six. From this list you will now be able to set your Value-Based Goals. I am now going to tell you exactly how to do that, and if you're not yet ready, come back to this section later. These goals really work – and feel good. You can see now why conventional weight-loss methods didn't work for me. When I got out the tape measure so that I could record inch loss round my waist, I remained totally uninspired. Of course I did, because the method I was using didn't reflect any of my values – Feel Good, Loveliness, Inspire and Sensual. Based on my values, however, my goals are –

- To feel full of energy when I wake up (Feel good).
- To go out with my husband knowing I look great (Loveliness).
- To write a book on my experiences to help others (Inspire).
- This one is a secret (Sensual)!

Now take a moment or two to write down your own value goals. Remember, they are not set in stone, so don't be afraid to try them out or change them.

Once you have identified your core values, you can set your goals incorporating these values as I described earlier (see pages 33–5). We talked about setting SMART goals, and now we are now in a position to do that with the added magic ingredient of your values. For example, if one of your values is Loveliness, a more attractive goal for you could be: 'To fit into my new dress which I will wear to my daughter's wedding. I will have achieved this within one month. I know I will have achieved this because I will feel and look lovely.'

Notice how the goal is attracting completion rather than driving you towards completion. We can use our values as our 'Northern Star' to help steer us in the right direction. The energy we need to orient ourselves to our goals is much healthier and more sustainable than the fear-based, depleting energy we may have used before. These old methods are characterised by force (crash diets) and threats ('I'll look awful if I don't'), by struggle (self-denial) and neediness ('I want to be loved and admired'). There are plenty of others that I am sure you can supply.

I invite you to incorporate your core values into all areas of your life. You will attract opportunities and experience more moments of happy coincidence – effortlessly. Your body will slim to a sustainable level and your life will feel lighter in body, mind and spirit.

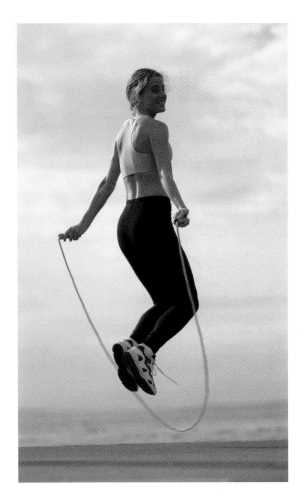

The Postures:
Part Six

18. Alternate Leg Forward Bend (Janu Sirsanana)

1 Sit with your legs stretched out in front of you, back straight and hands resting on your thighs.

2 Take hold of one of your feet and place it on the inside of the opposite thigh, so that the knee points out to the side.

■ Keep your back flat as though you have 'zipped up your spine'.

3 As you breathe out bend forward from the hips, sliding your hands down your outstretched leg to hold comfortably where you can. Hold for your 4–7 breaths.

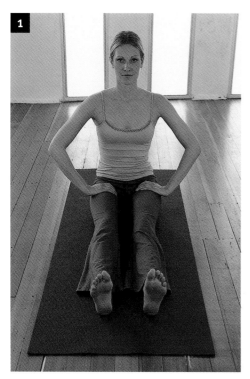

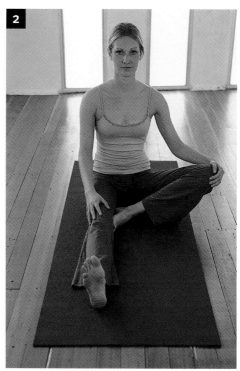

Benefits	
Body	Stretches and strengthens the hips/legs and back.
Mind	I stop tolerating it now.
Spirit	I honour my beauty within and without.

■ You can choose to use a sock, belt or scarf as a lever by wrapping it around the opposite foot and pulling on it to help you ease forward and still maintain a straight back (see picture 3a). Aim at directing your chin towards your shin rather than your head towards your knee, which will make your back rounded.

■ Repeat on the other side.

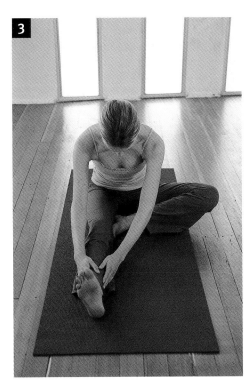

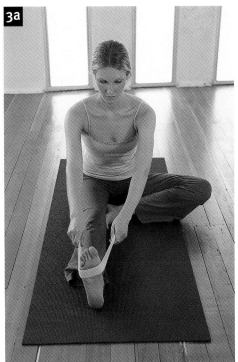

Benefits

Body	Optimises efficiency of the digestive system and stretches the whole of the back of the body.
Mind	It is safe to be vulnerable.
Spirit	Surrender to life's intelligence.

19. Forward Bend (Paschimottasana)

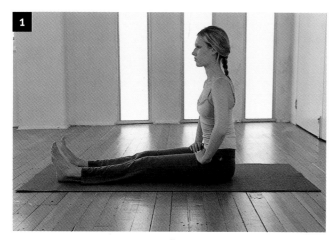

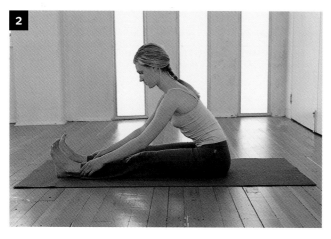

1 Sit with both legs outstretched and extend your spine (as though it is being 'zipped up' from the base to the neck). Rest your hands on your thighs.

2 Breathe in and on the out-breath slowly stretch your arms towards your feet as though your hips are a hinge. Move your chin towards your shins and clasp whichever part of your legs or feet you can with comfort. Use a belt if it helps you reach further (as in picture 3a on page 81).

■ Take up to 7 relaxing breaths; each time you breathe out, relax a little more.

■ Come up on an inhalation, working from the hips, sliding your hands up your legs. Your back is still straight. If you have any back challenges, to begin with walk your hands up your legs a step at a time to take the strain.

20. Balancing Calming Breath – Alternate Nostril Breathing (Nadi Sodhana Pranayama)

1 Sit or kneel comfortably (placing a cushion behind the knees between the thighs and calves if necessary), keeping the spine erect.

2 Gently bend your head forward a little and, using your right hand, place your right thumb over the right nostril and your right ring finger over the left nostril. Your index and middle finger are gently placed between and slightly above your eyebrows (see picture 2a).

■ Slowly breathe in through your left nostril, with your thumb closing your right nostril.

■ Pause gently, retaining the breath by closing both nostrils with the appropriate fingers, and when necessary exhale through your right nostril by releasing the thumb.

■ Breathe straight back up your right nostril, pause, closing both nostrils, and then exhale through your left nostril by releasing the ring finger. This completes one round of this wonderful calming breath.

■ Complete a couple at your own breathing rate to begin with, then work to the following pattern: breathe in for 2 counts (this makes it short and full), hold for the count of 8 (a long held breath) and out for the count of 4 – really pull your abdomen in and exhale every little last bit of air.

■ Perform 7 rounds. You will feel calmer and more balanced.

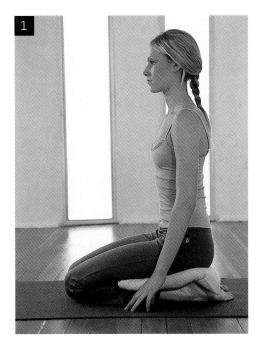

TIP – This breathing technique is fantastic for calming you in stressful situations (such as pre-exam nerves, flying, or an important occasion).

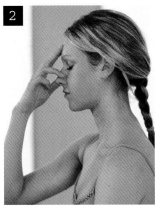
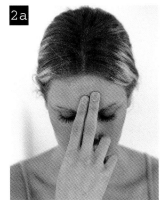

Letting Go

The best time to meditate is after your calming yoga postures, before you end your sequence with the relaxation exercise. If meditation is new to you, you can start with just 5 minutes and then gradually increase it to 20 minutes. If you prefer, you can omit the meditation now and do it at another time to suit you. This is the only part of the programme that you can take out of sequence.

Recharging the batteries

Meditation is one of the most beneficial practices I have discovered. It is where I commune with the highest part of myself and where I can gain perspective on my life. Meditation is so important and so simple, yet can often seem very difficult to the beginner. It is taken at many different levels and can have profound results. The simplest instructions I've heard are: 'Sit down and shut up' (meaning shut the senses up), but this is not as easy as it sounds.

In this chapter I describe five different meditations. You can try a new one each day, or the same one for a week or a month, then change if you wish. Many people stay, very happily, with the same meditation practice for years. If you find one that suits you and that supports you, then it's fine to stick with it – it's entirely up to you. Read through the instructions several times before you begin, or record them and play them back to yourself for the first few times you meditate until you are familiar with what to do. Remember too that it is important after your meditation to bring yourself slowly back to everyday wakefulness, especially if you need to drive somewhere.

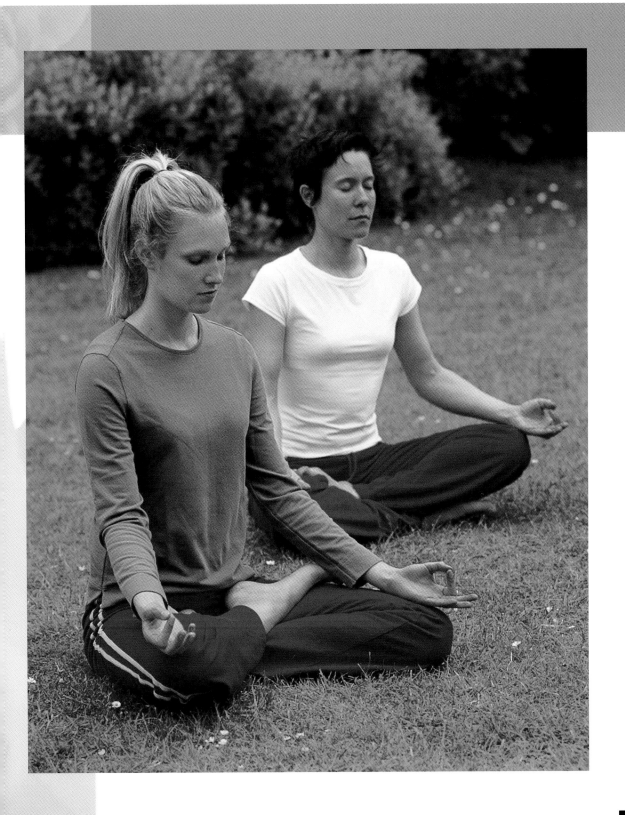

Meditation Postures

During meditation it is important that the spine is erect, so sit on the floor cross-legged on your mat, or on the edge of a hard cushion or foam yoga block. This tilts your pelvis forward slightly and helps to give you an ideal sitting posture. Alternatively, sit on a straight-backed chair. Place your hands in your lap, cupping your left hand in your right with your thumb tips touching. It helps to light a candle and to have it burning safely somewhere close by. I also have a shawl that I use just for meditation and when I put it on it helps me to connect with that peaceful part of me that I need to pass through in order to achieve the state of meditation.

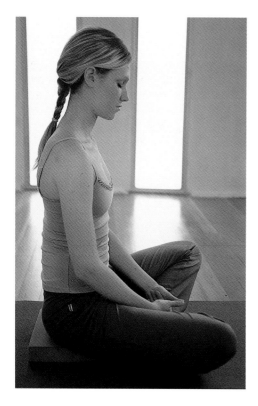

1. Slimming Meditation

Relax and close your eyes, take a few deep breaths and let go. As you exhale, imagine you are letting go of everything that you don't want or need that is connected with slimming. For example, that might be eating too much food, eating because of loneliness, boredom, happiness, or excitement, eating up the leftovers from the family's plates, or eating because it is there and provided for you.

■ It is time to release the overweight part of you, the part that doesn't feel good enough. It's as if your body has taken to wearing a bigger, heavier overcoat for this part of your life. Let's see what this overcoat of fat needs to say to us. Imagine taking it off and putting it on to an imaginary chair opposite you. Ask it some questions (perhaps something like: 'Why are you weighing me down?'; 'How best can I lovingly let you go, for I don't need you any more?'; 'What is it that you have come to teach me?'). Ask for your question to be answered within 24 hours, either now, in a dream, by symbols, by a thought, by a chance meeting with someone or by seeing a book with the answer. Believe me, you can learn through this 'overcoat'.

■ Now tell yourself that you release those old ways of eating and behaving, those old habits and patterns. Imagine that all your old ways, your old patterns and all the obstacles that prevent you achieving your desired size/weight are leaving your body, mind and spirit with each breath. You know that your spirit is perfect exactly as it is, and all you want to do is allow anything weighing you down to be released. Isn't it wonderful to know that there is a place inside you that is divine, perfect and at peace? Every time you release a breath, and release a little of your old belief patterns, you create more space inside you for something new.

■ After doing this for a few minutes, begin to imagine that every time you inhale you are breathing in *prana*, that wonderful life-force of the universe, and see it as a golden light. Within this life energy is everything you need and desire: a healthy, well-toned body, loving yourself no matter what, hands that put just the correct amount of nourishing food on the table, a powerful voice that says 'No' to foods that sabotage your regime, a head that shakes, saying 'No' to so-called friends and family who try to divert us from our visions and goals. Breathe all of that in with each inhalation. Imagine a new you and way of living opening up to you, not only slim, but alive, vital,

energised and yet at peace, connecting with your soul and spirit. See your life exactly how it would be if you had everything you desired; see, taste and smell it. In other words, what sort of colours would you see, how would you feel, how would you be emotionally? So let's let go of the old you and start to be the new you. It would be good if you could give the old you a name, and then think of a name to express the new you. For example, Stuck Suzie could transform into Supremo Suzie, Loser Lizzie into Lithe Lizzie, Victim Vivian into Vibrant Vivian. In my case it was Servile Celia to Successful Celia. By labelling something you can then identify it, and therefore rectify it and watch out for it in case it threatens to jeopardise your future plans.

■ Start to return your breathing to normal, feel your feet firmly on the ground, or your buttocks if you are sitting on the floor, open your eyes and come back to everyday consciousness. You are now in the process of creating a new you and a new life for yourself.

2. Purifying Meditation

Close your eyes and just imagine that a little candle flame is moving through your body. Start at the feet and work up each foot and leg, then up your body, arms, neck and head. This is the candle flame of purification, burning away unwanted, negative emotions; you could also imagine this flame burning away unnecessary fat and speeding up your metabolism. When you have completed the visualisation, sit quietly and let your thoughts go. Just be present, with the feeling of being there, at peace with yourself and the world. Bring yourself back to everyday consciousness by taking a few deep breaths, and feel your feet firmly on the ground.

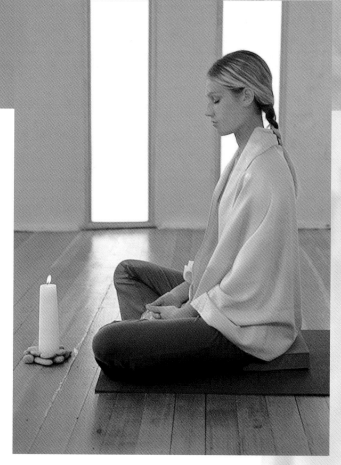

3. Meditation for When You Feel Stuck or at a Plateau With Your Weight

Begin by admitting your feelings and what is bothering you, how hard you feel you are struggling and yet somehow not achieving the results that you would hope for at this present time. Ask for help in knowing the way forward for you – how you can learn from your experience, how you can love yourself more, just as you are. Exactly what is the lesson in all this for you, and how can you grow through it and then move on? Then ask for some angelic help and see this in any way that helps you. One way that helps me is to see these lovely, friendly angels come along with 'fat magnets' and they give me a 'spiritual liposuction'. Feel the magnets go all over your body, paying particular attention to your fat-prone areas; allow the excess fat to be drawn out, effortlessly and lovingly. See yourself as you want to be, slim and vibrant. After 5–10 minutes, give thanks for any help received and bring yourself quietly back to everyday consciousness. This is done by taking a couple of deep breaths, feeling your feet firmly on the floor and perhaps looking at some different colours in the room.

4. Protection Meditation

I've heard it said that sometimes overweight people use their weight as a form of protection. The message they give themselves sounds something like: 'If I stay fat I won't have to face...,' and if this is true for you then Protection meditation will help. All of us have days when we feel more vulnerable than usual, and this is a lovely meditation to do at those times to increase our sense of self-worth and safety. I have used this meditation frequently, often squeezing it in at an odd moment at places of work by taking a few minutes in a lunch or coffee break, or by locking myself away in the loo – a wonderful place to take a quick 5-minute meditation at work.

■ Sit in your usual position with your spine erect. You are going to form a protective cocoon around you, so as you breathe in imagine breathing a protective shield up the right side of your body from below your feet. Pause in your breathing at the top of your head, and as you breathe out, form this protective shield down the left-hand side of your body, to the place where it began at your feet. Do this 7 times in total, each time expanding it out a few centimetres from your body so the cocoon becomes bigger each time. Now do the same from the bottom of your feet but this time up the back of the body. Pause at the top of your head and breathe out down the front of your body to the feet. Do this 7 times in total. You are then in your protective cocoon. Keep this image with you in challenging situations and with challenging people throughout your day.

5. Pink-bubble Worry Meditation

Worry often makes us overeat. Use this simple meditation in your allotted meditation time or at any time to help let your worries go. Think of a situation or problem that you have pressing on you at the present time. You have done everything you can to alleviate the problem, but it's still there, gnawing away at you. In your mind, see the problem, then in your imagination see it encased in a pink bubble and let it drift off into space. If the problem returns, do it again, and again, until you are free. Often I find that the situation improves when I yield it up like this.

Relaxation and Visualisation Exercises

When we are overweight often we seek comfort, and overeat as a reflexive response to this. Let's learn a new method – one that is not fattening! This technique will help you to recognise the various levels of tension that you experience through the day and will help you to unwind and avoid using food to help you relax and feel good. If you prefer, you may find it easier to record the instructions for this section and play them back while you do the exercise.

1 Lie comfortably on the floor – you can put a pillow or bolster under your knees for support if you wish. Cover yourself with a blanket (your temperature drops considerably in deep relaxation), and rest your head on a block a few centimetres thick – an average-sized telephone directory is ideal. You must make sure that you will not be interrupted, as to be disturbed abruptly from deep relaxation is unpleasant and can be quite a shock to your system. So hang a notice on the door, switch off your phone and relax. Have your feet about 45cm (18in) apart, with the toes relaxing outwards and your hands a little way from your body with the palms uppermost. We will use a sure, tried and tested method to relax our bodies: tensing and relaxing.

2 Breathe in and tense up the right leg by flexing the foot, lifting the heel a few centimetres off the ground, curling up the toes and taking the tension right up to your leg by

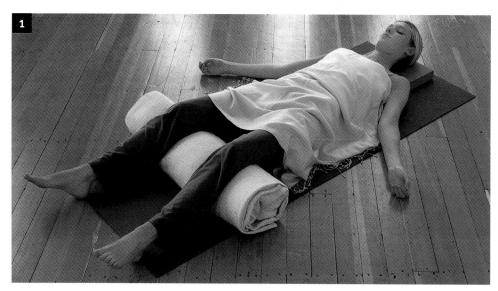

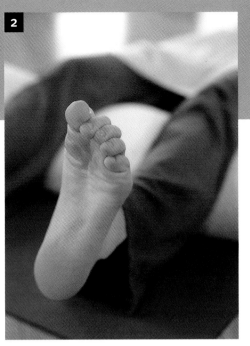

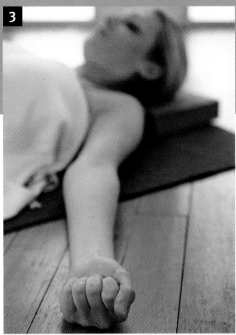

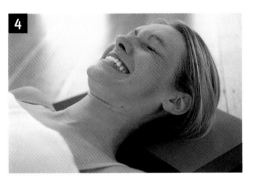

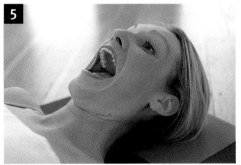

tensing the muscle in the right thigh. Hold the tension, and then as you exhale, release the breath together with the tension, letting the right leg relax completely. Breathe in and repeat on the left leg. Feel how relaxed both legs are.

■ Now turn your attention to your buttocks, and breathe in and squeeze the buttock muscles, pause, breathe out and relax the buttocks completely.

3 Breathe in and tense the right hand by making a fist and tensing along your arm up to your right shoulder, lifting it up to your ear; hold and release, completely letting go. Breathe in and repeat on the left arm.

4 Finally, the face, where we hold so much tension. Breathe in and tense, screwing up your eyes, clenching your teeth.

5 If you feel angry, open your mouth and utter a silent scream, then relax. Now breathe in and tense the whole body, hold, then relax and let go. You should feel soft and relaxed all over.

■ Now in your imagination take yourself to a beautiful tropical island. You can create an actual picture in your mind or just an impression or feeling; both are fine. See yourself lying on the beach, on warm, white sand. There are palm trees nearby, sending just enough soothing breeze to cool you, there are tropical birds singing in the distance and there are wonderful, colourful and exotic flowers; notice their scent, and absorb their healing perfumes into your body. The flowers have a magical aroma that cleanses, purifies and heals your body and mind of the need to overeat, so breathe the perfume into your body as if it is your own special aromatherapy cocktail, magically mixed especially for you. This will heal you and to help you to become whole again, become the lithe, slender, happy, creative person you were destined to be. The sun is shining down on your body, adding extra energy, healing and warmth where needed. Wow, do you feel good! When was the last time you felt so good? Right now you feel so relaxed and so empowered, listening to the soothing sound of the waves.

■ Now imagine your body as you would really like it to be. Please, be realistic and honest. How soft would you like your skin to be? What size waist and hips would you feel good with? How do you see your proportions? A little more muscle tone here and there? How about a lovely bone contour around your shoulders, a slim neck and slender hands and feet? All this is within your power to attain – in most cases, it will just mean calling on the three Ps (Persistence, Practice and Patience), but isn't it worth it? Don't you feel so sensual and good

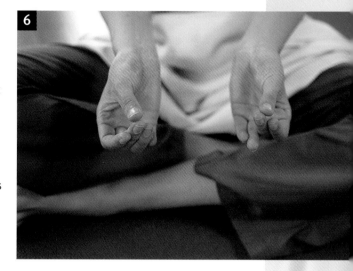

6

about yourself now? Aren't you going to get more out of life, being like this? You will radiate such good health and confidence that you are even going to make those around you feel good. Isn't it worth trading in that extra food or drink for this? You didn't even really enjoy it, did you? What trade-offs are you going to make in order to succeed in life? In silence, name one or two to yourself now, but make them small at first, so they are easy to attain.

6 Anchor this feeling by taking each thumb to the tip of your middle finger and gently stroke down this middle finger once, leaving the thumb at the base of the finger. This will have anchored this positive state in your body and mind, and it will be your own special, secret, slimming *mudra*. You can use this *mudra* at any time when you are feeling disempowered and need to bring yourself back to this state.

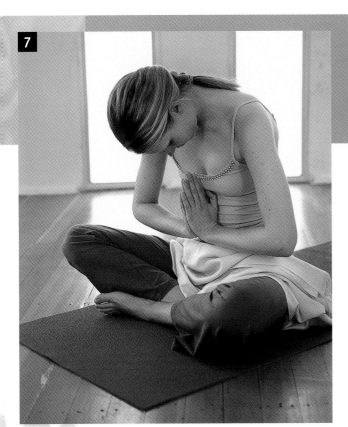

7

■ It's time to leave our tropical island now, and our relaxation session. You have revitalised your body, mind and spirit, each cell benefiting from this process, so that your whole body will work more efficiently. Gently, in your own time, wriggle your fingers and toes and have a good stretch; come back to everyday consciousness with confidence in yourself to achieve what you want in life.

To Conclude your Yoga for Weight Loss Session

7 Put your hands together in the gesture of prayer, the *namasté mudra*. Honour yourself for doing the regime and your willingness to achieve your goal. Honour yourself for who you truly are – a divine spirit and absolutely perfect just as you are now. And say to yourself: *namasté*. Well done. Well done. Well done.

GETTING MOVING

In addition to your daily yoga session, it would be helpful if you could also include some aerobic activity. What I suggest is very simple, but hugely effective.

■ Twice a week take a walk. Start gradually and then build up the pace so that you perspire. After 5 minutes' walking, start to become aware of your breathing pattern, and begin to synchronise your breathing with the steps you are taking. Breathe in for 4 steps, hold the breath for 2, breathe out for 4 and hold the out breath for 4. (Under no circumstances should this make you feel breathless, or dizzy – STOP IMMEDIATELY if this happens.) You should feel clear-headed and energised.

■ If this becomes too easy you can up the breathing to 6:3:6:3. Keep the breathing to about 10 minutes, and for the last 5 minutes of your walk, breathe normally. You can visualise the breath as that fat magnet, searching out unnecessary fat, and as you breathe out, breathe the fat out.

Eat to Energise

What if I were to give you a fantastic, extremely valuable thoroughbred racehorse that you knew would win races for you and make you a lot of money? How would you feed it? Would you give it carbonated drinks, coffee, junk food, grass-flavoured convenience foods, oats that had all the good bits removed, or perhaps chocolate-coated hay, as well as a few alcoholic drinks? Would you expect this wonderful creature to be performing at its best if you did this? No, of course you wouldn't. You would realise that it was a great investment and you'd spend time and money making sure that this fabulous winning machine was properly nourished to keep it in prime condition. So... if you'd do this for a horse, why on earth don't you do it for yourself? You are your own thoroughbred racehorse; you are far more valuable in terms of your potential – what you can achieve, and what you can contribute to the world around you – aren't you?

From now on, think of yourself as a great investment and be determined to bring out the best in yourself. That means only putting into your body food and drink that enhance your performance, give you vitality and richness of life and support your need and desire to succeed, not only in your Yoga for Weight Loss programme but also in your life in general.

'Yes, yes, YESSSSSS!' you say, but isn't the whole nutrition issue a complete muddle? It can be very confusing when one food company promotes a particular eating plan, but then you soon find that their advice is contradicted by another company, and the media run new stories about food scares and fad diets every day. I used to be confused too. I just didn't know what to eat, when to eat, how much to eat or how to eat it. But puzzle no more; let's take a common-sense, holistic approach, which will bring you energy and vitality.

Back to basics

We can do this by going back to the traditional wisdom of yoga. This can truly help us to make sense of eating and to understand how we need healthy food to achieve and maintain a lean, healthy body. No, don't worry; it's not about carbohydrates, fat percentages and grams of this or that. This is good basic information which is vitally relevant to us now and will help us reverse the trend towards obesity that is affecting so many of us in the

Western hemisphere. Briefly this can be summed up in a familiar phrase: 'You are what you eat.' So, if you eat highly processed foods, which are alien to your body, your digestion will be less efficient and this will result in you being lethargic, dull and fat. Simple.

Yogis divide food into three main groups. These are called the three *gunas*, or 'forces of nature'. Everything that has been created, be it animal, vegetable, mineral, or a feeling, condition or thought, is represented by a *guna* or combination of *gunas*. Each represents a different mood.

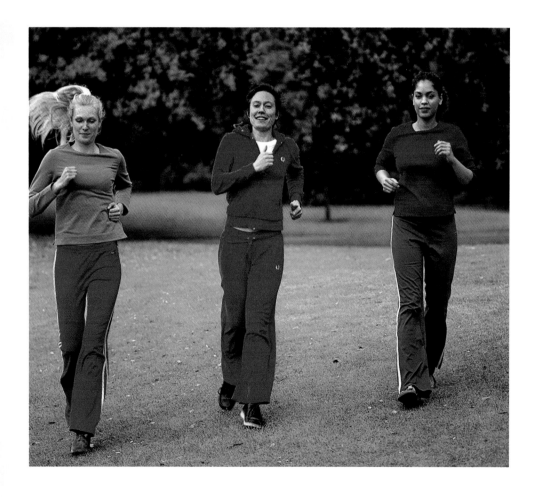

THE THREE GUNAS

Tamastic foods

These foods produce feelings of heaviness, dullness and lack of energy; they will cloud your thinking and contribute to a tendency towards depression. They will make you feel tired and stop you achieving in life, and lower your body's resistance to disease considerably. Tamastic foods include meat, battered fish, eggs, alcohol, overcooked foods, leftovers reheated, fried or barbecued foods, cakes and biscuits made with white flour, ice cream, sweets, white bread, refined, processed and pre-packaged foods, tinned foods, stale and tasteless foods, as well as anything containing preservatives or additives. In order to feel fully alive you must strictly limit the amount of Tamastic foods in your diet.

Rajastic foods

These foods have the opposite effect: they make you hyper and jumpy, so that you become more stressed and also more prone to circulatory and nervous disorders. They include coffee, tea, heavily spiced and salted products, flavoured crisps and peanuts, chocolate and carbonated drinks. Cigarettes and any other stimulant are also classed as Rajastic.

Sattvic foods

Foods in this group will calm the mind and body, make you vital and happy, and help to promote a long, healthy life. They are pure foods that are delicious in themselves. Once you have re-educated your taste buds not to expect heavily processed, salted and flavoured foods you will automatically start to enjoy natural flavours. Sattvic foods are organic and not genetically modified. So in this group we have fresh and dried fruits, freshly squeezed juices, raw or lightly cooked vegetables, salads, fresh fish, whole grains, nuts, seeds, sprouting seeds, wholemeal breads, honey, fresh herbs, herbal teas and organic dairy products. Nowadays we tend to overdo the dairy products, the majority of which are derived from animals that have been given hormones and antibiotics. So eat fewer dairy products as a first step to better health. In particular, avoid cheese because it is highly concentrated and has lots of fat in it. If you really want to lose fat, then cut out cheese altogether. On top of that, dairy products tend to produce more mucus in the body and I've noticed that since cutting down I have fewer colds. All Sattvic foods are easily digested, which means that you will have more energy for the good things in life.

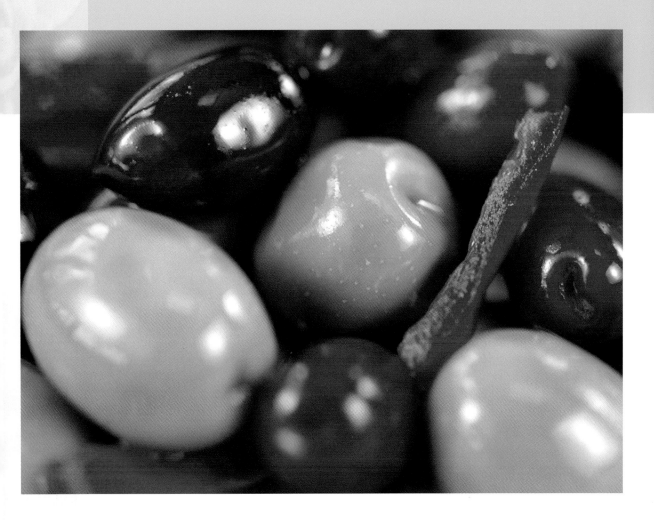

So it's very simple, really: if you want to feel clear-headed, full of energy and slim you choose foods from the Sattvic group. Of course there will be times when you indulge in a little something from the other groups, but before you do, ask yourself: 'What will be the consequences?' and if you are willing to accept them, then go ahead. Remember, the choice is yours.

The best way of giving things up is to lose the longing for them. Believe me: if you really pay attention to your diet you will get to a point where you do not want to drink so much coffee or alcohol, or eat so much meat. I remember 22 years ago, when I attended my first yoga class, I said: 'I will never give up meat.' Well, I just lost the taste for it, so giving it up happened quite naturally without me having to force myself to go without.

TIP – The more you put into a project, the more you get out of it.

SOME GUIDELINES TO SUPPORT YOUR PROGRAMME

■ Be calm when you eat – and this means no TV.

■ Put on some inspiring yet relaxing music and light a candle if possible. This will improve your digestion, which in turn helps you to lose weight and keep it off.

■ Always chew your food well. Boring, I know, but this will also help your digestion.

■ Personally I always give thanks for my food as well as thanking the people who have cooked it. I don't make a big deal of this. If I'm in company where it is accepted then I can do it out loud, probably with them, but if not I do it silently.

■ Do not eat after 7pm. Of course occasionally you will have to, and that is fine. But in the main run of things, you need to sleep well and not on a full stomach.

■ Eat some raw foods every day, preferably organic (but do wash them carefully). If you can't buy organic, rinse fruit and vegetables in a special cleansing wash available from health food stores.

■ Before each meal do the Hungry Test: sit down, put your hand on your tummy and gauge how hungry you are from 1 to 10, 1 signifying ravenous and 10 not hungry at all. You should aim always to be 3, 2 or 1. Towards the end of each meal, put your hand back on your tummy and gauge yourself again. You should aim to be a 7 or 8, not full up. If you are full to bursting, how can you expect your system to work efficiently? It won't, and the residue will be fat – on your body.

■ Only eat when seated and fully aware of what you're doing. This tip alone, strictly adhered to, will save you many added kilograms of fat. In fact it could save you 3kg (7lb – yes, half a stone) a year, just because of one new habit. Doing this, and achieving it, will help your resolution to eliminate other unhelpful habits.

■ Take time over your meal, since it takes 15–20 minutes to feel the effects of eating. Slow down and slim down.

■ Spread your food out on your plate; it looks as if you are eating more.

Take all the above points seriously but do not make yourself a slave to them. Enjoy your food but remember that it is there to serve you, not for you to serve it.

TIP – Nothing breeds success like success. Think of your achievements as building blocks that support future successful efforts.

A word on chocolate

Chocolate is one third saturated fat. Giving up chocolate – except on rare occasions – is a good thing. You already know that chocolate is full of sugar and fat and I won't bore you with the effects of this, but on the psychological side the great advantage of giving up a regular fix of chocolate is that you will be able to see objectively what it is that is lacking in your life that is pushing you to take that 'fix'. And the good news is that when you see what this void is in your life, you can take steps to fill it. So, in rejecting chocolate you are choosing sustainable happiness and doing yourself a big favour.

Keep it moving

Your system needs to work well, and that means having regular bowel movements. If you become constipated you feel and look bloated; it can give you headaches, or you can just feel out of sorts. If your body is working efficiently you should have a bowel movement every day. This can be encouraged by ensuring that there is plenty of fibre in your diet and if necessary taking 2 teaspoons of psyllium husks per day in a glass of water (drink immediately, then drink another cup of water directly afterwards). Or you can buy a product called Colon Cleanse which is available from all good health food shops and through internet mail order. This contains psyllium husks, cleansing herbs and

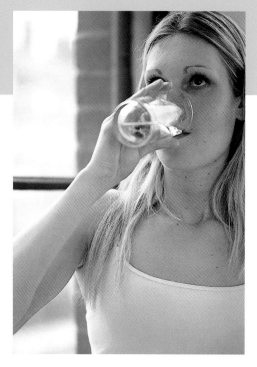

acidophilus to regulate the good bacteria in your colon as well as providing essential fibre. If you are not eliminating waste properly and regularly then your body can become clogged with residual faecal matter. This prevents you from digesting your food properly and you can gain weight just from your system's inefficiency. Many years ago, when I underwent a 33-day cleanse in California (under strict supervision), I had colonic irrigation as well, which completely clears out the colon, but even after 21 days of fasting, huge amounts of old waste were still coming out of my body. I have seen many wonders in my lifetime, but truly I was amazed! Apparently, according to the nutritionist, this is quite normal. But it's hardly surprising that my system was toxic and not working properly.

Fibre not only provides helpful roughage but also contributes to weight loss because it helps to satisfy our appetite. Fibre also steadies your blood sugar levels so you won't be so likely to feel desperate for a sugary snack.

Consequences

I will repeat that word: consequences. I want you to work with that word in your eating programme because it will help you understand and integrate the concepts I am advocating. Each time you eat something, ask yourself: 'What are the consequences of eating this?'

Let's look at an example. You are on Day 4 of your Detox and Eating Plan. You meet an old friend in the street and you pop into a local pub for a chat. He asks you what you would like to drink; you are excited and happy, and ask for a glass of wine. This is the point of decision. Stop for a moment and just think. What are the consequences?

1. You will stop the detox process.

2. You will risk jeopardising your initial grand weight loss – as well as being calorific, alcohol also encourages water retension.

3. That glass of wine may well lead to another and another. It will also give you an appetite for inappropriate food, because you associate salty, fatty snacks with alcohol, and because alcohol has the effect of destroying your awareness.

4. You may wake up in the morning feeling unwell (and probably hungover).

5. You will feel regret tomorrow that you failed in your resolve.

6. As you slipped in the first week, you will probably no longer believe that you will be able to complete the plan successfully.

7. Alcohol can affect blood sugar levels so that the next day you will crave sugary things.

So, is it worth it? If your answer is 'No', change your order to a sparkling water instead. What are the consequences?

1. You feel in control of your actions and therefore your life.

2. You wake up the next morning feeling energised and proud of your strength of will.

3. You will avoid weight gain through water retention.

4. You will feel more inspired to succeed in your endeavours to conquer fat once and for all.

5. Your whole body will feel healthier because your liver is not put under any extra strain.

Getting organised for success

1. Make sure you start your regime at a time that's good for you, so that you have the energy and opportunity to complete your goals.

2. Aim for the first week to have few or no social engagements that involve food.

3. Try to find extra time to relax and let the detox process take place, especially during the first week.

4. Enlist the help of your friends and family and tell them how they can support you. Better still, ask them to do it with you.

5. Plan how you will celebrate your success. What would really inspire and help you commit? A new outfit? A make-over? A balloon ride? Refer back to your values (see page 76) to help you decide what it is that would make the most powerful incentive for you. Be creative.

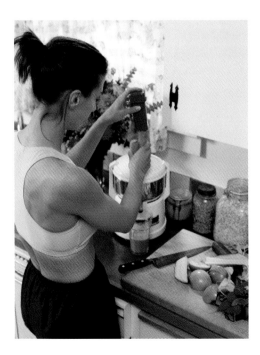

Shopping

You've heard it said before, but do be careful about going out shopping when you are hungry because that's when your resolve will be at its lowest. Some people find internet shopping helpful; why not try it if you tend to be swayed by supermarket special offers or the cheap deals of the day (which are usually very fattening)? Try these tips:

1. Always make a list and stick to it.

2. Don't go shopping hungry. Have something to eat first.

3. Always check the labels and don't purchase food with more than 5g (¼oz) of fat in it.

4. Don't walk down the confectionery aisles.

Preparing your food

1. Do it with love. Do it with love. Do it with love. Food cooked and prepared with love has a more beneficial energy than food cooked thoughtlessly or as a chore.

2. Make sure all your food is fresh, so that it contains the maximum quantities of vitamins and minerals. Vitamin C, for example, is very short-lived, so don't store fruit and vegetables for long periods.

3. Try to buy locally, and don't forget that it's good to eat foods that are in season.

4. Wash fruit and vegetables thoroughly. If you buy organic you don't need to peel them. Some

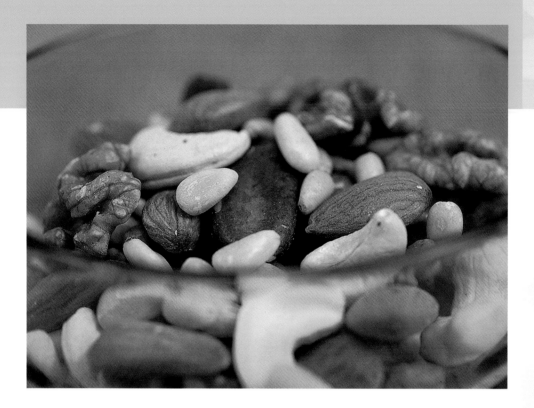

chemical sprays are poisonous, so if your food is not organic, try washing it with a special spray to remove pesticide residues (see Resources, page 140).

5. Wherever possible, eat your fruits, vegetables and nuts raw. If you can, have something raw at least once a day.

6. When cooking fruit and vegetables keep the cooking time to a minimum. They should, wherever possible, maintain their crunchy texture when cooked.

7. The way you cook your food is very important. Steaming is very good, as is low-fat grilling. If you decide to boil your food, use very little water and bring it to boiling point before adding the food. Reserve any remaining water for soups and stocks. Use a thick-bottomed, heavy, non-stick frying pan, or a wok for stir-frying. You will need only a very small amount of olive oil brushed across the bottom to stop the food sticking. Otherwise invest in a health grill, which will provide you with a low-cost way to cook without using fat. Think seriously about throwing out your deep-fat frying pan. This way of cooking is full of calories and can be the cause of dreadful burns and fires – is it worth it just because of the taste? If you follow my programme, you will find that you feel so happy inside that you no longer want the food you used to think of as a 'treat'.

8. Add seasonings to taste at the table, not in the cooking. There are some wonderful varieties available that make just plain salt and pepper seem very boring – see page 131.

Food at home

1. Clear your cupboards of anything that might tempt you to break your diet. That means banishing anything like biscuits, crisps or chocolate that you can get at if your resolve fails. Don't buy them. You are going to be No. 1 for a few weeks, and if other members of the family are desperate to have them, they can buy them themselves and keep them in their rooms. No exceptions.

2. Choose fresh fruit and healthy snacks. Pre-packed carrot batons are my standby.

3. Health food shop proprietors can be a mine of useful information on healthy eating, and many have attended courses on nutrition. They will usually give freely of their time. Many large stores also now carry information on healthy eating.

4. Start to make eating well a new, exciting hobby; educating yourself can be fun as well as informative. There are some great websites (see Resources, page 140), and there are often interesting food programmes on the TV and radio. You cannot overeducate yourself regarding your own health and well-being.

Adapting your own recipies

1. Recipes usually specify far too much fat. Just use a teaspoon of virgin olive oil brushed quickly over the food to be grilled or stir-fried; often you can cut it out completely.

2. Substitute skimmed milk for whole milk or semi-skimmed, and fromage frais or low-fat natural yoghurt for cream.

3. In all chicken recipes remove the skin.

4. Substitute stock cubes that can be high in salt and make your own healthy stock by using Marigold bouillon or miso.

5. Grill rather than fry, preferably in a health grill (see Resources, page 140).

6. If you are eating meat, cut the visible fat from it before you grill or dry-fry it.

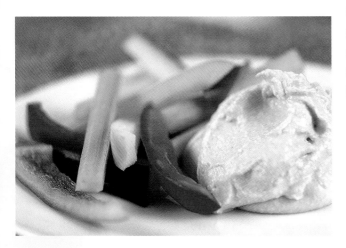

The 28-day Detox and Eating Plan

This eating plan will detoxify your system and help to re-educate your taste buds so that you are not always reaching for processed foods. Your digestive system will also have a chance to recover from overindulgence. You will find some of the recipes, including my own favourites, at the end of the chapter.

After the initial 7-day programme outlined below, you can go on for another 7 days, and then another and another, making 28 days in total – the choice is yours. During this time you will lose fat from your body, but more importantly your mind will become that of a permanently slim and healthy person through practising the personal development exercises. The first 7 days will be the strictest in dietary terms, and for this week I have set out a shopping list to help you prepare. It will also serve as a de-addiction course because you will no longer crave the foods that are most destructive to your body.

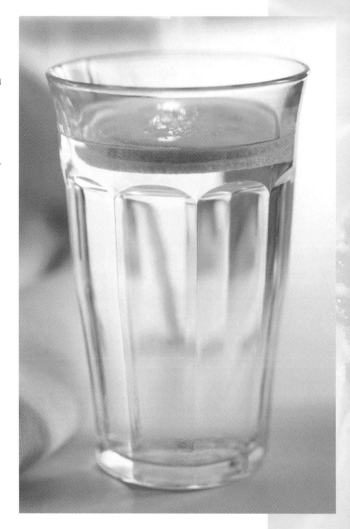

Week One

No coffee, tea or alcohol for the first 7 days. To drink you may have only filtered or bottled water and herbal teas. Each day on rising, drink one glass of hot water with the juice of half a lemon squeezed into it. Try to eat organic food wherever possible. No salt or other condiments should be added until specifically stated in the programme.

Shopping list

1 grapefruit
4 lemons
6 apples
6 bananas
Bottled water or a filter jug
Cereal and muesli (sugar- and salt-free varieties)
Wheat-free cereal
Skim milk and/or soya milk
Soup (low-fat, preferably organic)
175g (6oz) white fish
150g (5oz) green beans
75g (3oz) new potatoes
3 baking potatoes
1 packet of plain, unsalted rice cakes
3 packets of stir-fry vegetables
2 x 75g (3oz) cooked breasts of organic chicken (you can use Quorn fillets instead, if you are a vegetarian)
1 tuna steak (or chicken breast) to cook
1 can of tuna

Tofu (the best variety is silken tofu) from a health food store
Salad ingredients, including tomatoes — get a good variety
2 tubs of sugar-free fruit compote, store-bought or homemade (see page 115),
1 large tub of reduced-fat organic plain Greek yogurt
1 large tub of plain cottage cheese
1 small jar of low-fat mayonnaise
1 small can of organic baked beans (no-added-sugar variety)
Reduced-calorie bread
25g (1oz) pine nuts
Wholegrain rice
A variety of organic vegetables to make soups, but do not choose potatoes, parsnips, peas or lima beans for this, as they contain too much starch
1 packet of wheat-free crispbreads

For this first week, I have kept the food simple. This will enable you to spend more time and energy on your Yoga for Weight Loss programme, making sure you do your postures each day. Going on a healthy slimming programme takes a lot of time and effort; if you are spending hours in the kitchen, you will have less time for yourself. Do get your family's support; tell them how you are feeling and explain that you want to get healthy, slim and fit. Make it fun and interesting; perhaps with the promise of this new, vibrant mother/wife they will want to help out.

DAY 1
Breakfast
Half a ripe grapefruit (do not add sugar – you will soon learn to appreciate nature's sweetness). 25g (1oz) low-fat, unsweetened cereal with 150ml (¼ pint) skimmed milk (or low-fat soya milk for those who wish to cut down on dairy products).

Mid morning
1 piece of fruit (try to change the variety from day to day).

Lunch
175g (6oz) fish, steamed or grilled, with lemon juice. 150g (5oz) green beans. 75g (3oz) new potatoes cooked in their skins or 1 baked potato (never add butter to baked potatoes, and if eating out make sure you order one without butter).

Mid afternoon
2 plain rice cakes.

Evening meal
75g (3oz) organic chicken or 125g (4oz) tofu with stir-fry vegetables (if, for convenience, you purchase a pack from a supermarket, ditch the sauce).

DAY 2
Breakfast
Half a grapefruit. 50g (2oz) muesli with 150ml (¼ pint) of skimmed milk or low-fat soya milk.

Mid morning
1 apple.

Lunch
1 baked potato, filled with tuna mixed with low-fat mayonnaise, and fresh salad.

Mid afternoon
1 banana.

Evening meal
Home-made soup (see recipes, page 116, or choose one of your own; make it low in fat but high in vegetable content).

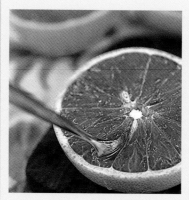

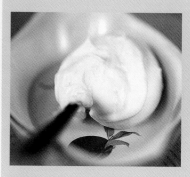

DAY 3
Breakfast
1 small tub of fruit compote (see recipes, page 115) mixed with half a 120g (4oz) tub of organic low-fat Greek yoghurt.

Mid morning
2 wheat-free crispbreads with Marmite or low-fat soft cheese.

Lunch
Organic chicken salad made with one chicken breast (skin removed), or Quorn fillets if you're vegetarian. Low-calorie or home-made dressing (see pages 125–7)

Mid afternoon
1 apple.

Evening meal
Organic baked beans on 2 slices of reduced-calorie bread (without spread).

DAY 4
Breakfast
1 apple, 1 banana.

Mid morning
2 rice cakes.

Lunch
Salad of 25g (1oz) nuts mixed with any raw vegetable or salad ingredients, plus apple horseradish dressing (see recipes, page 127).

Mid afternoon
1 banana.

Evening meal
50g (2oz) cottage cheese and 1 tomato on 2 wheat-free crispbreads.

DAY 5
Breakfast
Fruit compote or 2 pieces of fruit (not banana).

Mid morning
1 banana.

Lunch
Home-made soup of your choice.

Mid afternoon
2 rice cakes

Evening meal
1 small tuna steak or medium chicken breast, grilled. Unlimited fresh, lightly cooked vegetables (not potatoes, parsnips, peas or broad beans).

DAY 6
Breakfast
2 pieces of fruit.

Mid morning
1 banana.

Lunch
Cottage cheese in a baked potato with natural flavourings, such as herbs or Tabasco.
Fresh salad.

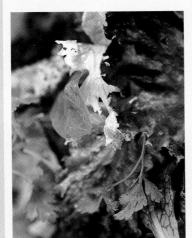

Mid afternoon
1 apple (if not having the baked apple after your evening meal).

Evening meal
Cooked wholegrain rice with chopped vegetables.
1 baked apple (if you chose not to have it earlier; see page 129).

DAY 7
Breakfast
25g (1oz) wheat-free cereal (available from health food shops) with 150ml (¼ pint) skimmed milk or low-fat soya milk, or porridge (see recipes, page 116).

Mid morning
1 small bowl of soup, home-made or a miso instant variety.

Lunch
Cottage cheese and vegetables (as a salad, if you like). Try to include sprouting beans.

Mid afternoon
2 wheat-free crispbreads.

Evening meal
Stir-fry vegetables with tofu or organic chicken, or a dish from the recipes section (see pages 121–5).

Week Two

At this point, some self-assessment is called for. How are you feeling? Lighter? You may have weighed yourself. If so, have you lost weight? I don't always recommend weighing, because one can become hooked on what the scales say and we all know that we women can put on kilos overnight due to water retention. Weigh yourself if you wish, if it helps you, otherwise go by your clothes and by an honest appraisal of yourself. Your clothes will fit better after this first week; you will have got over the initial feelings of discomfort from the detoxifying processes. In fact, you will feel raring to take on the following weeks. If you have experienced headaches for the first few days, don't worry: this is a natural consequence of your withdrawal from caffeine in tea and coffee.

We will be adding more to your food intake this week. Stick with the lemon juice and hot water on rising.

DAY 8
Breakfast
Half a grapefruit.
25g (1oz) organic cereal (sugar- and salt-free variety) with 150ml (¼ pint) skimmed milk or low-fat soya milk.

Mid morning
2 rice cakes – try the flavoured variety, they're delicious.

Lunch
Salad made with cooked wholegrain rice (about 75g/3oz) with chopped vegetables in a mayonnaise tofu dressing (see recipes, page 127). Or mix together 1 teaspoon olive oil and 2 teaspoons balsamic vinegar to make a dressing. Add plenty of ground dried herbs, or better still use chopped fresh herbs.

Mid afternoon
1 piece of fruit.

Evening meal
175g (6oz) fish, grilled, dry-fried or steamed, with oriental salad (see recipes, page 126).

DAY 9
Breakfast
Half a grapefruit.
Mushrooms (poached in a little milk or grilled) on 1 slice of wholegrain bread.

Mid morning
1 banana.

Lunch
1 pitta bread filled with home-made paté (see recipes, page 118) and salad, with a few olives if you wish.

Mid afternoon
2 wheat-free crispbreads with low-fat spread.

Evening meal
1 medium portion of lentil and buckwheat slice (see recipes, page 124) with cooked vegetables. If you have a health grill, use it to grill them for a change; try peppers, mushrooms and aubergines.

DAY 10
Breakfast
Porridge (see recipes, page 116).

Mid morning
2 pieces of fruit.

Lunch
1 baked potato with tuna and fresh salad.

Mid afternoon
1 wholegrain flapjack (home-made or from a health food store).

Evening meal
Cottage cheese and nut loaf (see Recipes, page 121) with steamed vegetables.

DAY 11
Breakfast
50g (2oz – uncooked wieght) quinoa cereal (cook and freeze half the portion for use next week).
3 tablespoons low-fat live yoghurt with 1 tablespoon linseeds sweetened with 1 teaspoon honey.

Mid morning
2 rice cakes (save these for lunch if you prefer).

Lunch
Organic raw vegetables with hummus dip (see recipes, page 119).

Mid afternoon
1 frozen banana – this can be prepared easily the previous day by peeling and placing in the freezer. It makes a delicious snack, tasting like banana ice-cream without the fat or the calories.

Evening meal
Vegetarian sausages (see recipes, page 121) with any green vegetables and swede. You can have a small amount of instant gravy if you wish.

DAY 12
Breakfast
1 thick or 2 thin slices of wholemeal bread spread with organic fruit spread (mango is delicious).

Mid morning
2 pieces of fruit.

Lunch
Fruity lentil soup (see recipes, page 117) with one bread roll. (Stick to 2 crispbreads or 2 oatcakes without wheat if you wish to keep wheat free.)

Mid afternoon
1 low-fat, low-sugar flapjack.

Evening meal
Pasta with cream cheese and cashew sauce (see Recipes, page 124).

DAY 13
Breakfast
Fruit compote (see recipes, page 115) with low-fat organic yoghurt.

Mid morning
1 low-calorie, low-sugar flapjack.

Lunch
2 soya and lentil burgers with salad (see recipes, page 122).

Mid afternoon
1 piece of fruit (alternatively, have a baked apple for your evening meal – see recipes, page 129).

Evening meal
Chick pea and spinach soup (see recipes, page 118).
Optional baked apple.

DAY 14
Breakfast
If you wish, have 1 boiled egg or 1 poached egg on wholewheat bread; otherwise have 1 slice of bread with honey or fruit spread.

Mid morning
1 banana.

Lunch
Pitta bread stuffed with feta cheese, 6 olives and salad.

Mid afternoon
Exotic fruit such as mango or papaya.

Celebration evening meal
Low-fat garlic mushrooms (see recipes, page 120).
Grilled tuna steak with steamed vegetables or salad.
1 frozen banana.

■ Congratulations! you are half-way through your programme. You will no doubt be feeling more alive, relaxed and confident. We have introduced eggs (optional) to your programme and have added some simple recipes. If you do not wish to use eggs in cooking you can get an egg substitute from health food stores.

Week three

DAY 15
Breakfast
25g (1oz) quinoa cereal (pre-cooked) with 150ml (¼ pint) skimmed milk or low-fat soya milk. 100g (3½oz) fruit compote (see recipes, page 115) with 1 tablespoon low-fat Greek yoghurt.

Mid morning
1 apple.

Lunch
Broccoli soup with 2 garlic toasts (see recipes, pages 116 and 120).

Mid afternoon
1 low-fat yoghurt.

Evening meal
Spinach and sweet potato casserole (see recipes, page 122).

DAY 16
Breakfast
25g (1oz) cereal with skimmed milk, or porridge (see page 116).

Mid morning
1 small packet of mini rice cakes.

Lunch
Red bean salad with 100g (3½oz) feta cheese or tofu (see recipes, page 125).

Mid afternoon
1 pear.

Evening meal
Vegetarian mushroom stroganoff (see recipes, page 123).

DAY 17
Breakfast
100g (3½oz) fruit compote (see recipes, page 115).

Mid morning
2 wheat-free crispbreads, any variety with low-fat spread.

Lunch
1 medium bowl of carrot and coriander soup with 1 bread roll or 2 rice cakes (see recipes, page 117).

Mid afternoon
1 banana.

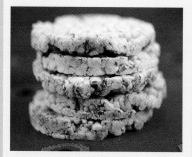

Evening meal
Pasta with cream cheese and cashew sauce (see recipes, page 124).

DAY 18
Breakfast
1 slice of wholewheat bread with sugar-free spread.

Mid morning
Mango and tofu dessert (see recipes, page 129).

Lunch
1 medium bowl of home-made or bought organic soup (less than 3 per cent fat) with 1 bread roll or 2 wheat-free crispbreads.

Mid afternoon
1 pear.

Evening meal
Chicken and vegetable stir-fry using 1 organic chicken breast, or Quorn fillet if you are vegetarian.

DAY 19
Breakfast
25g (1oz) cereal – try a new one for a change, with 150ml (¼ pint) skimmed milk or low-fat soya milk.

Mid morning
2 plums, if available, otherwise
1 apple.

Lunch
7x10cm (3x4in) piece of cheese
savoury slice (see recipes,
page 119).
Salad with alfalfa sprouts, tomato
and cucumber.
Low-calorie dressing of your
choice or apple horseradish
dressing (see recipes, page 127).

Mid afternoon
1 low-sugar, low-fat flapjack.

Evening meal
2 grilled Quorn burgers and a
salad of shredded white cabbage
with as many other salad
vegetables as you wish.
Salad dressing of your choice
(see recipes, page 125–7).

DAY 20
Breakfast
1 banana, 1 apple and 1 orange.

Mid morning
1 small packet of flavoured mini
rice cakes.

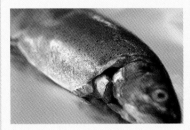

Lunch
1 baked potato with low-calorie
hummus (see recipes, page 119)
and lettuce and tomato salad.

Mid afternoon
2 wheat-free crispbreads with
slimmer's jam (see recipes,
page 115).

Evening meal
Grilled fish, steamed vegetables
and 1 small baking potato.

DAY 21
Breakfast
Low-calorie cereal of your choice
with 150ml (¼ pint) skimmed milk
or low-fat soya milk.

Mid morning
1 piece of tropical fruit.

Lunch
Sausage sandwich made of 2
Quorn sausages (or home-made

vegetarian sausages, see recipes,
page 121) cut lengthwise and put
between 2 pieces of low-calorie
bread. You can spread the bread
with mustard or a spicy sauce.

Celebration evening meal
Prawn cocktail made with 100g
(3½ oz) prawns, lettuce and
yoghurt dressing (see recipes,
page 126).
Vegetarian mushroom stroganoff
(see recipes, page 123).
Dried fruit mousse (see recipes,
page 128).

■ Well done, you have achieved
three weeks at your diet and yoga
programme.

■ Do this exercise NOW. Sit down,
take your right arm straight up in
the air above your head, bend it
at the elbow, and pat your back,
at the same time saying 'I'm
brilliant, I've done it.'

■ Think about how you actually
feel; have a look at yourself. Your
body will now be showing signs
of your discipline and dedication
to the Yoga for Weight Loss
programme.

Week four

DAY 22
Breakfast
Half a grapefruit.
1 slice of wholemeal bread topped with grilled mushrooms.

Mid morning
1 low-fat, low-sugar flapjack.

Lunch
Soup of your choice, either home-made (see recipes, page 116) or a bought low-fat organic variety.
1 wholewheat roll or 2 rice cakes.

Mid afternoon
1 piece of fruit of your choice.

Evening meal
Choose any dinner from the previous week (but not Day 21!).

DAY 23
Breakfast
Porridge (see recipes, page 116). Use water instead of milk if preferred.

Mid morning
2 wheat-free crispbreads with low-fat spread.

Lunch
Salad of lettuce, alfalfa sprouts, tomato and cucumber, a little dressing of 1 teaspoon olive oil and 2 teaspoons balsamic vinegar, 25g (1oz) pine nuts, 1 baked potato and 1 tablespoon hummus.

Mid afternoon
25g (1oz) dried fruit.

Evening meal
Choose any dinner from the programme so far.

DAY 24
Breakfast
100g (3¹/₂oz) fruit compote (see recipes, page 115) with 2 tablespoons low-fat Greek yoghurt.

Mid morning
1 small packet of corn cakes or rice cakes.

Lunch
Tuna-stuffed pitta bread (see recipes, page 118).

Mid afternoon
1 apple or pear.

Evening meal
Choose one from the previous weeks.

DAY 25
Breakfast
2 slices of bread with low-sugar spread of your choice.

Mid morning
1 apple.

Lunch
1 medium bowl of carrot and coriander soup with 1 garlic toast (see recipes, pages 117 and 120).

Mid afternoon
1 low-fat, low-sugar flapjack.

Evening meal
Chicken salad made with 1 chicken breast (skin removed), lettuce, tomato, cucumber, alfalfa sprouts and any other of your favourite salad vegetables, with a low-calorie dressing. Use Quorn instead of chicken if you are vegetarian.

DAY 26
Breakfast
100g (3¹/₂oz) fruit compote (see recipes, page 115) with silken tofu or 2 tablespoons low-fat Greek yoghurt.

Mid morning
2 rice cakes.

Lunch
Soup or salad.

Mid afternoon
1 pear.

Evening meal
Grilled fish of your choice with a large plate of vegetables (including 1 small baking potato or 3 small new potatoes).

DAY 27
Breakfast
Choose any breakfast from the previous weeks.

Mid morning
Mixed fruit salad.

Lunch
Baked potato filled with hummus or red bean salad (see recipes, pages 119 or 125).

Mid afternoon
25g (1oz) dried fruit.

Evening meal
2 vegetarian sausages (see recipes, page 121) with green vegetables and swede, and some instant gravy if you desire.

DAY 28
Breakfast
Dried fruit mousse (see recipes, page 128) served decadently in your best dish.

Mid morning
A tropical fruit or your favourite variety.

Lunch
7x10cm (3x4in) piece of cheese savoury slice with a salad of your choice, and apple and horseradish dressing (see recipes, pages 117 and 127).

Mid afternoon
1 small packet of mini rice cakes.

Celebration evening meal
Prawn cocktail made with lettuce, 50g (2oz) prawns and low-fat seafood dressing (see recipes, page 126).
Grilled chicken or fish with steamed vegetables.
15cm (2in) portion of date and rhubarb cake (see recipes, page 129). If you have a birthday cake candle, put it on top to celebrate your achievements.

■ You have worked through 28 days of my Yoga for Weight Loss programme. Fantastic! You will be looking and feeling better. You will feel like a different person – in fact you *are* a different person. You will have made major internal 'shifts' which, because of your insights and self-discoveries, are permanent. You will have acknowledged and let go of emotional/mental fat as well as body fat. You will have learned and experienced the wonderful consequences of eating healthy foods.

■ Practising your daily yoga, following the Yoga for Weight Loss programme and completing the personal development exercises will have transformed you into somebody beyond your wildest dreams. You will be slimmer, have more energy, feel sexier, more confident, calmer, more loving and clear-headed, and your life will be effortless and full of joy. Well done!

■ You can work through the programme again, repeat a favourite week or start to investigate some new healthy recipes and integrate them into this programme.

Yoga for Weight Loss Recipes

I know you will love these recipes, all of which I use regularly. The whole family can enjoy these beautiful, healthful and tasty dishes, and you can serve them at dinner parties or save them for romantic meals with your partner. All you need to do is change your style of cooking to a healthy one, which will fill you and those around you with energy! Cooking the Yoga for Weight Loss way will give you the opportunity to enhance other people's lives as well as your own.

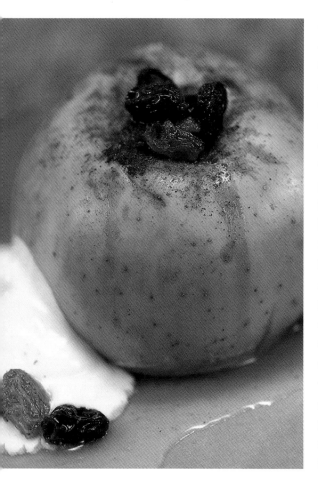

Serving instructions

Always present your food beautifully. I have served some dinner-party disasters attractively and managed to get away with it. Choose pâté dishes for their shape and colour; a silver salver always looks fantastic. Earthenware complements healthy food very well; and have you ever tried serving food in fruit? A rice dish presented in a dug-out half pineapple looks fabulous. The main idea is to give the impression that you are special and that your food is special. Make the table look attractive. Light candles. A meal is an occasion. I also choose complementary music, such as vibrant Latin American music if I'm having Mexican food or sitar music for an Indian meal. Create a good atmosphere and feed yourself on that. We've come across illusion dressing — well, now we've got illusion eating. With a little thought and planning, you can convince yourself that you are eating at the most exclusive restaurant and that you are the most wonderful person in the world — which, of course, you are.

Breakfast

Home-made muesli
Serves 6–8

Make this up at the beginning of the week, keep it in an airtight container and it will last you through to Day 7.

500g (1lb) mixed grains. If you are avoiding wheat just use oats, barley flakes and maize flakes
2 tablespoons chopped mixed nuts
2 tablespoons raisins or sultanas
1kg (2lb) chopped dried fruit such as dates or papaya

1. Mix all the ingredients together and store in an airtight container in a cool dark place.

Slimmer's jam
Makes 10–12 servings

1 sugar-free fruit jelly
250–500g (8oz–1lb) fresh fruit, lightly cooked

1. Make up 600ml (1 pint) of sugar-free jelly according to the instructions on the packet.
2. Add the fruit.
3. Mix together and store in jam jars. This will keep for two weeks in the refrigerator.

Fruit compote
Serves 6

This keeps well in the fridge and is great served with low-fat organic Greek yoghurt.

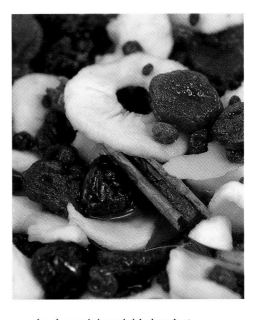

75g (3oz) unsulphured dried apricots
75g (3oz) dried apples
75g (3oz) dried prunes
40g (1½oz) sultanas
40g (1½oz) raisins
425ml (¾ pint) natural unsweetened apple juice
6cm (2½in) cinnamon stick
Thinly pared rind of unwaxed lemon

1. Chop the prunes, apples and apricots into smaller pieces, put all the fruit into a bowl and cover it with the apple juice.
2. Put in the cinnamon stick and lemon rind. Leave the fruit to soak for 12 hours.
3. Remove the lemon rind and cut it into thin strips. Put the fruit, cinnamon stick and lemon rind into a saucepan. Bring gently to the boil over a low heat. Simmer for 15 minutes.
4. Discard the cinnamon stick and serve hot or cold.

Pete's porridge
Serves 2

My husband has had this for breakfast nearly every day for 20 years, and he's the fittest person I know!

50g (2oz) oats
2 medium banana, chopped
Water or milk

1. Place the oats in a bowl and add the banana.
2. Stir in the water or milk, or a combination of both, up to just above the level of the oats.
3. Microwave on full power for 3 minutes and stir before serving.

Soups

Broccoli soup
Serves 4

1 teaspoon sea salt
700ml (1½ pints) filtered water
500g (1lb) broccoli, broken into florets and the stalk chopped into small pieces
Grains of Desire (see page 131), for seasoning
Chopped fresh mixed herbs, for garnishing

1. Put the salt and water into a large saucepan. Bring to the boil, add the broccoli, cover the pan and simmer for 10 minutes.
2. Remove the broccoli from the pan with a slotted spoon and put it in a food processor with a little of the cooking water. Reserve the remaining water.
3. Blend the broccoli for 2–3 minutes, until very smooth.
4. With the processor still running, gradually pour in the rest of the broccoli water.
5. Season with Grains of Desire and garnish with herbs.

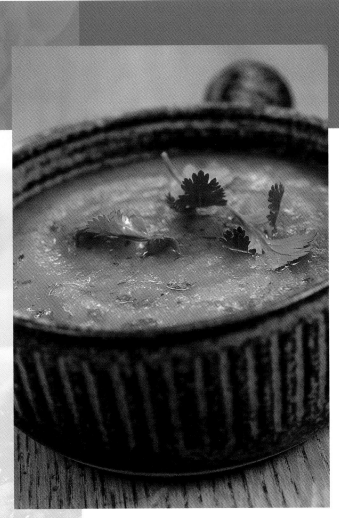

1. Place all the ingredients, except the miso, into a large saucepan, reserving some coriander as a garnish. Bring to the boil and then turn down the heat.
2. Simmer for 25 minutes, until the vegetables are soft. Liquidise until smooth and return to the pan to keep hot.
3. Mix the miso with a little of the soup in a blowl and add to the pan. Season and garnish with some fresh coriander to serve.

Fruity lentil soup

Serves 4

50g (2oz) dried split red lentils, washed
50g (2oz) dried apricots
1 large potato, roughly chopped
1.2 litres (2 pints) stock made from purified
  water and Marigold bouillon
1 teaspoon black mustard seeds
Juice of 1 small lemon
1 teaspoon ground cumin
Seasoning

1. Put the lentils and apricots in a large saucepan. Add the potato and the remaining ingredients.
2. Bring to the boil, then cover and simmer for 30 minutes. Cool and liquidise.
3. Reheat and adjust the seasoning to serve.

Carrot and coriander soup

Serves 4

1 litre (1¾ pints) vegetable stock
1 large onion, chopped
750g (1½lb) carrots, chopped
1 fresh red chilli, de-seeded and chopped
Juice and grated rind of 1 lemon
1 garlic clove, peeled
Seasoning
1 bunch of fresh coriander, chopped
1 tablespoon miso

Chick pea and spinach soup
Serves 4

A lovely meal in itself. You can use watercress instead of the spinach if you prefer.

2 teaspoons virgin olive oil
1 large onion, chopped
2 garlic cloves, crushed
50g (2oz) dried split red lentils, washed
50g (2oz) long-grain rice, rinsed
1.8 litres (3 pints) filtered water
Seasoning
100g (3½oz) dried chick peas, soaked overnight and simmered for 1 hour or until soft (why not make a double quantity and freeze for future use?) or 1 x 400g (14oz) tin, drained
1 large bag of spinach leaves, washed

1. Heat the oil, add the onion and garlic, and cook for about 4 minutes, until golden and soft.
2. Add the red lentils and rice, water and seasoning (you will need a little sea salt) and simmer for 15 minutes.
3. Add the chick peas and spinach, and simmer for another 5 minutes. Adjust the seasoning if necessary and serve hot.

Snacks

Tuna-stuffed pitta bread
Serves 2

100g (3½oz) button mushrooms, sliced
2 tablespoons chopped fresh parsley
2 tablespoon low-fat yoghurt
Squeeze of lemon juice
100g (3½oz) tinned tuna (in brine, not oil)
2 large wholemeal pitta breads

1. Add the mushrooms and parsley to the yoghurt. Stir well.
2. Flavour with the lemon juice and seasoning and stir in the tuna.
3. Halve the pitta breads, warm the halves under a grill and stuff them with the mixture.

Red bean pâté
Serves 2

1 x 200g (7oz) tin red kidney beans, drained
100g (3½oz) extra-light soft cheese
1 tablespoon Bragg's Liquid Aminos (see page 131)
A few sprigs of fresh parsley

1. Simply put all of the ingredients into a food processor and mix together.
2. Serve attractively in a small pâté dish and garnish with a few sprigs of parsley.

Hummus

Serves 2

Good old hummus. This can be used as a dip, for sliced mixed vegetables or as a great filling for a baked potato.

100g (3½oz) dried chickpeas, or
  1 x 400g (14oz) tin chickpeas, drained.
1 garlic clove
3 tablespoons low-fat plain yoghurt
Juice of 1 lemon
1 tablespoon tahini (a paste made with
  sesame seeds)
Seasoning
2 tablespoons chopped fresh parsley

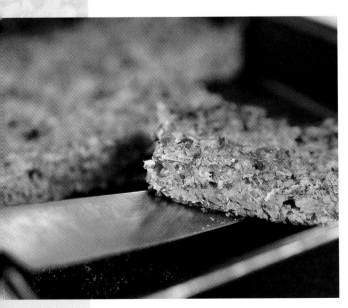

1. If using dried chickpeas, soak them in water overnight. Drain, place them in fresh cold water and bring to the boil. Simmer for 1–2 hours until tender. Drain. You don't need to do this if using tinned.

2. Put the chickpeas into a liquidiser or food processor with the garlic, yoghurt, lemon juice and tahini and process until smooth. Season to taste, sprinkle with fresh parsley and serve.

Cheese savoury slice

Serves 4

75g (3oz) low-fat hard cheese, finely grated
2 large carrots, finely grated
1 small onion, finely grated
½ green pepper, finely grated
1 egg, beaten
150g (5oz) rolled organic oats (use the
  cheaper, softer ones)
50g (2oz) organic butter, melted
1 teaspoon Marmite
Seasoning and chopped fresh herbs to taste

1. Preheat the oven to 190°C /375°F/gas 5.

2. Mix all the ingredients together, making sure they are well blended.

3. Press into a greased Swiss roll tin and bake in the oven for 20 minutes. Cut into slices and leave to cool before removing from the tin.

Garlic toasts

Makes 4

Garlic bread is a wonderful treat, but loaded with calories. Try this delicious alternative instead.

4 medium slices of wholemeal bread
2 garlic cloves, cut in half
Freshly ground black pepper

1. Preheat the grill
2. Toast the bread slices on both sides. Whilst they are still hot, rub each piece of toast with a cut garlic clove and season with black pepper.
3. Serve at once.

Low-fat garlic mushrooms

Serves 2

4 large flat mushrooms
100g (3½oz) low-fat soft cheese
2 garlic cloves, chopped
1 tablespoon chopped fresh parsley, plus
  extra for garnishing
2–3 teaspoons low-fat soya or skimmed milk
Seasoning

1. Wash the mushrooms, then arrange them, stalk side down, in a microwave or on a grill and microwave for 3 minutes or grill for 4–6 minutes.

2. Put the soft cheese into a mixing bowl and add the garlic, parsley and milk, beating until smooth and creamy.
3. Turn the mushrooms over and divide the soft cheese mixture between them. Level off the surface, patting around the stalks (if the stalks are too long just trim them a little), and season.
4. Grill until lightly browned and bubbling, or microwave for another minute.
5. Add some sea salt, freshly ground black pepper and a little chopped parsley to taste.

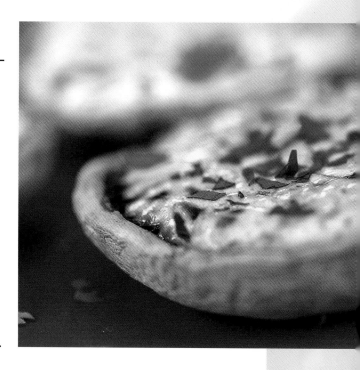

Main courses

Cottage cheese and nut loaf
Serves 6

1 teaspoon virgin olive oil
225g (7½oz) tub low-fat cottage cheese
2 free-range eggs, beaten
3 celery sticks, finely chopped
50g (2oz) raisins
50g (2oz) walnuts, chopped
1 level tablespoon tomato purée
2 tablespoons low-fat soya milk
50g (2oz) rolled oats
Seasoning

1. Preheat the oven to 190°C/375°F/gas 5.
2. Brush the inside of a 500g (1lb) non-stick loaf tin with the olive oil.
3. In a bowl, mix the cottage cheese with the beaten eggs, celery, raisins, walnuts, tomato purée and milk.
4. Stir in the rolled oats, season the mixture and turn into the tin.
5. Cover with kitchen foil and bake in the oven for 30 minutes or until the loaf is firmly set. Turn out when cold. Serve with a salad.

Vegetarian sausages
Serves 4

100g (3½oz) dried split red lentils or
  yellow split peas, washed
1 medium carrot, grated
1 medium onion, grated
450ml (¾ pint) filtered water
175g (6oz) medium oatmeal
1 tablespoon virgin olive oil
100g (3½oz) fresh wholewheat breadcrumbs
2 garlic cloves
1 teaspoon Marmite
1 tablespoon tomato purée
1 teaspoon chopped fresh thyme
1 teaspoon chopped fresh sage
1 tablespoon chopped fresh parsley
Seasoning
Flour for coating

1. Put the lentils or split peas in a saucepan with the carrot and onion . Add the water and bring to the boil, then simmer for around 20 minutes.
2. Add the oatmeal and cook for a further 10 minutes. Remove from the heat and stir in the remaining ingredients. Leave to cool.
3. Shape into sausages and roll in flour. Fry in a minimum amount of oil, or barbecue or grill, for about 10 minutes, turning regularly.

Soya and lentil burgers

Serves 4

2 tablespoons virgin olive oil

4 large celery sticks, finely chopped

2 medium onions, finely chopped

1 garlic clove, finely choped

125g (4oz) dried soya beans, soaked, cooked
  and finely chopped

125g (4oz) dried green lentils, soaked,
  cooked and finely chopped

600ml (1 pint) stock

1 teaspoon curry powder

Seasoning

4 tablespoons chopped fresh mixed herbs

100g (3½oz) wholewheat flour

1 free-range egg, beaten

50g (2oz) wholewheat breadcrumbs

A little oil for shallow frying, or use a
  health grill

1. Heat the olive oil in a saucepan, stir in the celery, onions and garlic, cover and cook gently for 10 minutes.

2. Mix in the soya beans and lentils and cook, stirring, for 2 minutes.

3. Add the stock and curry power and season well. Bring the mixture to the boil, cover and gently simmer for 45 minutes, until all the liquid is absorbed and you have a light, fluffy purée.

4. Take the pan from the heat, beat in the herbs and let the mixture cool.

5. Add enough flour to be able to form the mixture into approximately 10 patties, about 1.5cm (¾in) thick. Coat them in beaten egg and then in breadcrumbs.

6. Heat a little oil in a pan and fry until golden brown on both sides or put on a preheated health grill and cook until well done. You could also barbecue the burgers.

Spinach and sweet potato casserole

Serves 4

1 teaspoon virgin olive oil

1 large onion, chopped

2 garlic cloves, crushed

2 tablespoons tomato purée

1 medium sweet potato, peeled and diced

1 x 400g (14oz) tin tomatoes

1 x 400g (14oz) tin chick peas, drained, or
  100g (3½oz) dried chick peas, soaked
  overnight and cooked for 1–2 hours until soft

1 large bag of spinach leaves, washed

1 tablespoon miso

Seasoning

1. Brush the oil over the bottom of a large pan and heat. Add the onion and garlic and cook, stirring, for 4–5 minutes. Add the tomato purée and stir well.

2. Add the sweet potato, tomatoes and chick peas to the saucepan. Bring to the boil, then

reduce the heat and simmer gently for 30 minutes until the sweet potato is tender.

3. Add the spinach leaves to the saucepan and cook gently for 3–4 minutes, until the leaves have wilted. Stir thoroughly.

4. Add the miso to a little of the cooking liquid in a bowl and stir until well mixed. Put this mixture back into the pot, stir, and serve immediately.

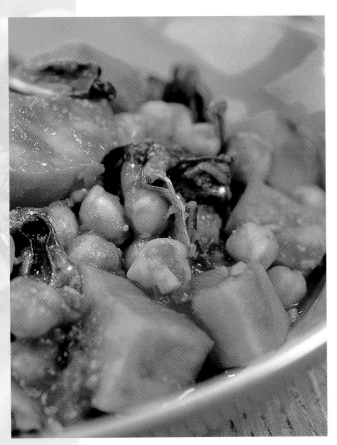

Vegetarian mushroom stroganoff
Serves 4

1 teaspoon virgin olive oil
500g (1lb) leeks
2 garlic cloves, crushed
500g (1lb) button mushrooms, or a
  medley of button and exotic varieties
1 heaped tablespoon plain wholemeal flour
125ml (4fl oz) vegetable stock made with
  Marigold bouillon
1 teaspoon Dijon mustard
1 teasoon tamari sauce or Bragg's Liquid
  Aminos (see page 131)
1 bay leaf
Seasoning
150g (5oz) tub low-fat plain organic yoghurt

1. Heat the oil in a large non-stick saucepan and sauté the leeks, garlic and mushrooms for 5 minutes until soft.

2. Add the flour and cook for 3 minutes more, stirring all the time so it doesn't catch, then gradually add the stock and stir until the sauce thickens.

3. Add the mustard, tamari or Liquid Aminos, bay leaf and seasoning.

4. Simmer for 1 minute, then add the yoghurt. Discard the bay leaf and serve immediately.

Lentil and buckwheat slice

Makes 4–6

Delicious served hot with vegetables, or cold as part of a packed lunch.

100g (3½oz) buckwheat
1 teaspoon virgin olive oil
1 medium onion, chopped
1 medium carrot, chopped
175g (6oz) dried split red lentils, washed
900ml (1½ pints) vegetable stock
2 tablespoons chopped fresh parsley
1 teaspoon dried mixed herbs
1 teaspoon Marmite
Seasoning

1. Preheat the oven to 200°C/400°F/gas 6.
2. Toast the buckwheat in a hot frying pan until brown (there is no need to add fat). Heat the oil in a saucepan and sauté the onion and carrot until the onion is transparent.
3. Add the buckwheat, lentils and the remaining ingredients. Bring to the boil, reduce the heat and simmer for about 30 minutes, until all the liquid is absorbed.
4. Press the mixture into a greased 25cm (10in) flan tin, and bake in the oven for 30 minutes.

Pasta with cream cheese and cashew sauce

Serves 2

I like this meal because the cauliflower bulks it out and fools me into thinking I am eating loads of pasta. The nutty taste also satisfies my craving for nuts (too many of which can be fattening).

50g (2oz) pasta shells
Sea salt
175g (6oz) cauliflower florets
175g (6oz) carrots, sliced
175g (6oz) button mushrooms, sliced

For the sauce:
2 tablespoons crunchy cashew butter (peanut
  butter will do if you can't get cashew)
120g (4oz) low-fat soft cheese
8 tablespoons skimmed milk or low-fat
  soya milk
Seasoning
Finely chopped fresh herbs for garnishing

1. Boil the pasta in salted water according to the packet instructions, drain and keep warm.
2. Boil the cauliflower, carrots and mushrooms in a little water so they steam-cook as much as possible, or use a steamer if you have one.
3. To make the sauce, mix together the cashew or peanut butter, low-fat soft cheese and milk.

4. Bring to boil over a low heat, stirring all the time. Add the mushrooms and simmer for 1–2 minutes. Stir the pasta and vegetables into the sauce, season to taste and garnish with herbs.

TIP – If you are not too great at sauce-making, you can put it in the microwave rather than boiling it. It's much simpler and doesn't catch.

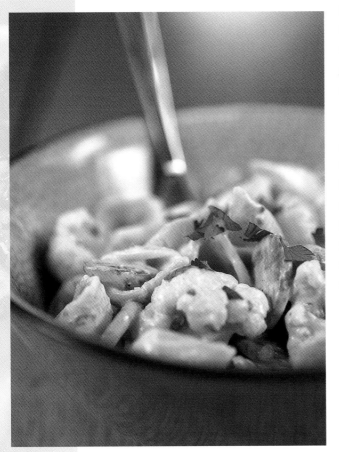

Salads and dressings

Red bean salad
Serves 4–6

175g (6oz) dried red kidney beans, soaked
  overnight and cooked for about 1½ hours,
  including 10 minutes' hard boiling, or use
  2 x 400g (14oz) tins, drained
1 onion, finely chopped
1 garlic clove, crushed
1 tablespoon red wine or balsamic vinegar
3 tablespoons virgin olive oil
1 tablespoon tomato purée or sugar-free
  tomato ketchup

1. Preferably with the beans still hot, simply mix all the ingredients together, turning the beans well so that they are all coated.
2. Leave for at least 2 hours to marinate, giving them an occasional stir.
3. Use this on its own or as a base for a main meal, adding celery, sprouts, sliced mushrooms or whatever you fancy and have to hand.

Oriental salad
Serves 3–4

½ Chinese cabbage, chopped
1 green pepper, chopped
1 red pepper, chopped

For the dressing:
1 tablespoon chopped stem ginger
2 tablespoons tomato purée
1 teaspoon chopped fresh coriander
1 tablespoon virgin olive oil
1 tablespoon good-quality balsamic vinegar
Freshly ground black pepper to season

1. Mix the ingredients for the dressing together.
2. Toss the vegetables and dressing together and serve chilled.

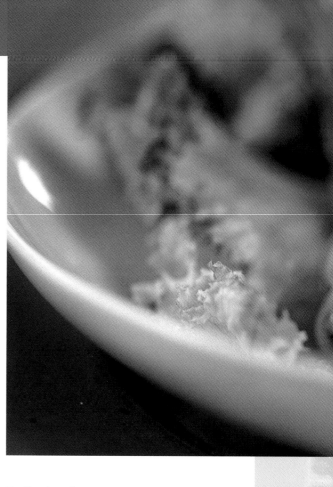

Seafood salad with yoghurt dressing
Serves 4

The dressing in this recipe is also ideal for a low-calorie prawn cocktail.

A selection of mixed salad leaves, such as cos, frisée, lollo rosso, little gem, watercress and radicchio
500g (1lb) mixed seafood (such as prawns, mussels, squid, crab and scallops)

For the dressing:
1 tablespoon tomato purée
1 garlic clove, crushed
2 tablespoons low-fat Greek yoghurt
2 drops Worcestershire sauce
2 teaspoons lemon juice
Seasoning

1. Whisk all the ingredients for the dressing together and pour over the leaves and seafood.
2. Season to taste and serve chilled.

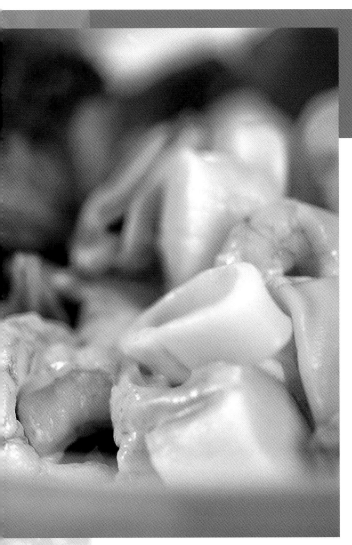

Slimmer's nectar salad dressing
Serves 2

4 teaspoons organic apple cider vinegar
2 teaspoons miso (any variety)

1. Stir the cider vinegar into the miso and
mix well.
2. Leave the mixture as it is or add one of the
following to spice it up: chopped fresh basil;
the juice of ½ orange plus 1 teaspoon grated
rind; the juice of ½ lemon plus 1 crushed
garlic clove.

Dairy-free mayonnaise

Serve with salads, as a topping for a baked
potato or for delicious home-made coleslaw.

75g (3oz) natural tofu
1 tablespoon low-fat organic yoghurt
1 tablespoon white wine vinegar
1 teaspoon grainy Dijon mustard
1 garlic clove (crushed, if you are not using
a blender)

1. Put all the ingredients in a blender and blend
until smooth, or mix well in a bowl.

Apple horseradish dressing
Serves 2–3

2 eating apples
2 tablespoons lemon juice
225g (7½oz) low-fat crème fraîche
2 teaspoons horseradish sauce

1. Coarsely grate the apples and simply mix
all the ingredients together and serve.

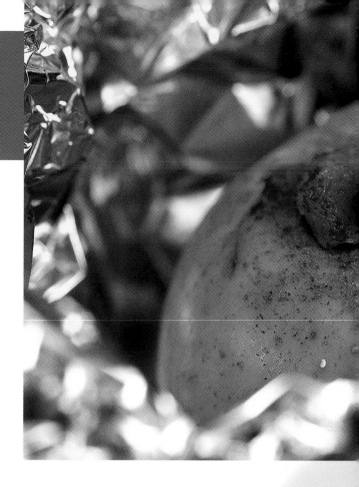

Desserts

Dried fruit mousse
Serves 4

100g (3½oz) dried prunes
100g (3½oz) unsulphured dried apricots
1 litre (2¼pints) fresh orange juice
300ml (½ pint) filtered water
15g (½oz) gelatine or agar-agar for
*   vegetarians*
2 free-range eggs, separated
Low-fat natural Greek yoghurt

1. Put the prunes, apricots and orange juice into a bowl and leave them for 12 hours.
2. Soak the gelatine in a small pan in 4 tablespoons of the orange juice.
3. Stone the prunes and put the prunes, apricots, remaining juice and filtered water into a blender and blend them until you have a smooth purée.
4. Put the purée into a saucepan and set it on a low heat.
5. Melt the gelatine gently over a low heat, and then quickly stir it into the fruit purée. Beat in the egg yolks and stir until the mixture is very thick and creamy, without letting it boil. (But note that if you are using agar-agar, bring it to the boil and let it cool slightly before adding the egg yolks.)
6. Take the pan from the heat and let the mixture cool until it is on the point of setting. Stiffly whip the egg whites.
7. First fold the yoghurt and then the egg whites into the fruit mixture. Pour the mousse into a large bowl or individual dishes and put into the fridge to set. Decorate creatively – express yourself!

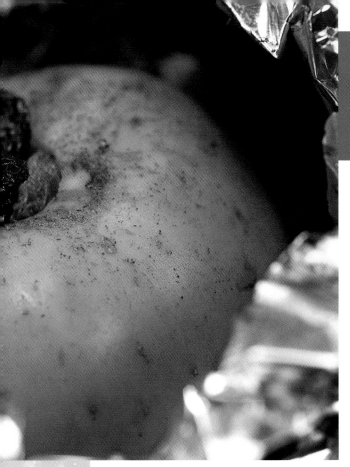

Mango and tofu dessert
Serves 2

1 ripe mango
100g (3½oz) silken tofu

1. Peel the mango and chop the flesh.
2. Process the mango and tofu in a food processor until you have a thick, smooth purée
3. Serve chilled in individual glasses.

Date and rhubarb cake
Serves 6

175g (6oz) self-raising wholemeal flour
75g (3oz) organic butter
100g (3½oz) Demerara sugar
100g (3½oz) chopped dates
225g (7½oz) uncooked rhubarb, sliced
1 egg, beaten with 4 tablespoons skimmed milk

1. Preheat the oven to 180°C/350°F/gas 4.
2. Rub the flour and butter together, then add all the other ingredients and beat well.
3. Place the mixture in a greased cake tin and bake in the oven for 1–1½ hours, or until golden. Delicious served warm with low-fat plain yoghurt.

Baked apple
Serves 2

2 baking apples
Handful of sultanas and raisins
2 tablespoons apple juice
½ teaspoon ground cinnamon

1. Preheat the oven to 200°C/400°F/gas 6. Core the apples and stuff with the sultanas or raisins.
2. Place each apple on a square of foil, pour over the apple juice and sprinkle with a little cinnamon. Make into parcels with the foil.
3. Bake in the oven for about 15 minutes until the apple is soft. Serve with a little low-fat organic Greek yoghurt or fromage frais.

A Word On...

Sprouts

They're ridiculously cheap, highly nutritious, easily grown in any home, extremely low in calories, and believe it or nor they actually taste nice as well! This wonder food is the humble sprout. No, not the Brussels kind, but the sort you get with Chinese meals. There are about 20 different types of beans, seeds and grains that you can sprout. As they can be grown on your window-sill they stay completely fresh until you eat them and you know that no harmful sprays have been used on them. They are very versatile and can be used in so many ways: for instance, you can add bean sprouts to bread dough; use sprouts as a sandwich filling instead of lettuce or tomato; add sprouts to scrambled eggs or omelettes; stir them into soups or casseroles at the last minute; add them to meat-loaf or rissole mixtures; or simply enjoy them in salads.

Growing them couldn't be simpler. Enlist the children's help – they will love it, and it will support you in your healthy-eating drive. An ideal sprout to start with is alfalfa (obtainable from any health food shop). Then you'll need a jam jar (or similar), some sort of porous material to put over the top (a clean kitchen cloth would be ideal), and an elastic band to secure it. A 500g (1lb) jam jar will house about 1 dessertspoon of seeds. Check your seeds over and take out any odd bits or broken ones before you put them in. Stand the jar in a fairly warm place. Rinse the seeds twice daily with warm water, giving them a little shake, but be sure to empty all the water out, draining well. They mature in about 4–5 days. It couldn't be easier – so come on, get sprouting! You can also get electric sprouters that allow you to grow a wider range (see Resources, page 140).

Miso

This is a brown seasoning paste available in tubs or small plastic bags. It is made from fermented whole soya beans, sea salt and, in some kinds, whole grains such as barley or brown rice. It is high in protein and contains B vitamins, is natural and can be used instead of stock cubes. There are several types available and perhaps the best one to start with is *Hugo* miso, made simply from soya beans. *Mugi* miso contains barley; it is lighter in colour and slightly less salty in flavour. *Kome* contains white rice and is very salty, while *Genmai* is made with brown rice and is slightly sweet. Miso is very concentrated, so you need add only a little to soups and casseroles. You put it in at the end, just before serving, never during cooking as this destroys the nutrients. If the miso is a stiff variety you take about a dessertspoonful of it, put in your serving dish, add a little of the liquid from your soup and mix it around to dilute it, then add the rest of your soup.

Tofu

Tofu is soya bean curd. It is extremely low in calories and lends itself to a variety of dishes, sweet and savoury. It is fairly bland on its own, but can be marinated or stir-fried with tamari (or good-quality soy sauce). The best sort is silken tofu.

Seasonings

Don't limit yourself to salt and pepper. Go mad and expand your seasoning range. Try this one: Fruits Alfresco, which has sun-dried tomatoes, black pepper, roasted garlic, olives, sweet peppers, red onion, basil and wheat grass, all in a handy grinder. Or what about Grains of Desire, which is said to spice up your sex life?! This has black peppercorns, nutmeg, cloves, orange rind, red rose petals, grains of paradise and ginseng. Information on how to obtain these is given on page 140.

If you can't get fresh herbs, then organic dried ones are a good substitute. Fiddes Payne produces mixed dried organic herbs in a handy grinder, and these release a wonderful aroma.

Bragg's Liquid Aminos is another healthy way of seasoning, and provides an alternative to tamari and soy sauce. It has a delicious savoury flavour, and contains 16 different amino acids. It is available at health food stores.

Use these seasonings after cooking. That way you individualise the taste of your food.

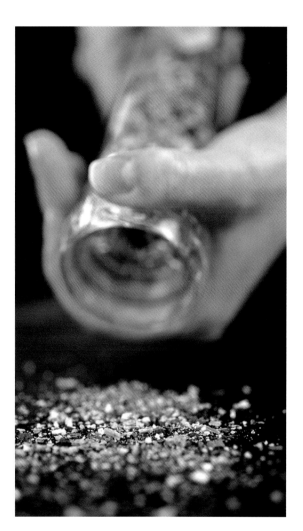

Power Boosting Tips

There are times when, no matter how well your programme is going, extra stresses put pressure on you. This is when you are more likely to slip. Below I have listed a few of the ways in which I have helped my students and clients cope with those unexpected 'blips'. Read them now, before you have need of them, then you will be prepared!

Staying aware, and alert!

A constant physical reminder that you have committed yourself to the Yoga for Weight Loss programme will help you combat temptation. In my classes I hand out a key ring and I suggest each of my students attaches it to the zip of their handbag or purse as symbol of all the good things that are now within their grasp. The key ring will serve as a constant reminder that they have made a conscious choice to change, become more positive and release their weight problems. So find a symbol that can inspire you, amuse you, or just remind you that what you're doing for yourself is really important. Much more important than reaching for that sugary treat or bar of chocolate.

The following are some of my instant power-boosting tips for when it feels as if your will-power might be slipping. Before you trot off in search of some comfort food, you can try these.

If you want to nibble – try this first:

Slimming Breath

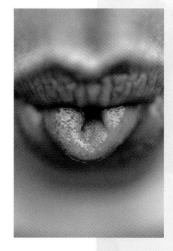

- Stick out your tongue, its sides folded upward to form a sort of channel or tube, and then breathe in slowly and deeply through your mouth.
- Withdraw your tongue and place it behind the upper teeth for a short time, with the breath retained, before exhaling slowly through both nostrils.
- The exhalation should be longer than the inhalation.

Good to use if you are desperate to snack because it appeases hunger and thirst.

Slimming *Mudra*

- Any time you need a psychological slimming boost, simply perform your slimming *mudra* (see page 93). This will bring back your feelings of empowerment and motivation.

If you are upset or frustrated – don't eat, try this first:

Cleansing Breath

• Sit crossed-legged on the floor, and imagine you are blowing out an imaginary candle in front of you.

• Imagine you are blowing out those blocks that in the past have prevented you from losing weight and sticking to a healthy eating regime.

• Bend forwards as you exhale forcefully through your mouth and then pull in your tummy on the final breath to get the last bit of breath out. This is good for removing the tension that comes with anger or frustration.

If you are really angry, here's an idea:

Exorcising Breath

• Find a quiet place where you won't be disturbed.

• Using a cushion or pillow, pound out all your aggression.

• Do this for about a minute, shouting and screaming and really letting go.

Yoga is not all about contemplating your navel, it's about being real. If you are angry, be aware of it and get it out before it becomes destructive to you or those around you.

Powerplus visualisation for specific weight-loss goals

Create a mental picture of your chosen goal. Something you aspire to, something you really want, such as being slimmer, fitter, on the beach or swimming on holiday. See it in as much detail as you can, with colour, movement and sounds. Make it specific. Hold it for a while and then allow it to fade. Now create a mental picture of your present situation or 'current reality' – you, as you are now. See this too, in full detail, not hiding anything from your awareness, then allow it to fade.

Now imagine you are looking at a large cinema screen split into two halves, Allow the image of your current reality to form in the left half and the vision of your goal to form in the right half. Hold them both on the screen together. In this way you are creating structural tension, which will seek to be resolved. Now say to yourself the following affirmation: 'I choose to have or be... [your goal].' Now imagine a flow of energy from the picture on the left of the screen to the picture on the right. Focus all your attention on the right-hand picture. Tell yourself that you WANT this to be your future. Make a statement to yourself that you BELIEVE it will come true.

FAQs

I hope that my book has helped to answer most of your questions about yoga and reducing. Some questions seem to crop up all the time, and here are a few of them; but do let me know if you have any more.

Q Should I drink water on this regime?

A Always drink water, preferably eight glasses a day. It cleanses the system and helps prevent hunger. In fact, often when we feel hungry we are actually thirsty, so when the hunger pangs strike, try drinking a large glass of water first.

Q Yoga is not an aerobic exercise, so how can I lose weight?

A Aerobic exercise will help you to lose weight and to maintain weight loss. What I am advocating, however, is that you start to be aware of the food that you eat and the reasons why you eat it. I build up your 'choice muscles' so that before you eat anything you are aware you are doing it. How many times have you eaten without really deciding to, as though the cake had a mind of its own? Most weight-reduction programmes fail because we lose control. Yoga for Weight Loss puts you back in control and makes you aware of your actions. It's better to exercise on effective eating rather than exercise to try to burn off the effects of eating. It

takes a lot of exercise to burn off one chocolate bar — surely if you exercise to stop yourself eating the chocolate bar in the first place, that must work better for you? I wholeheartedly support aerobic exercise, but do it for enjoyment and health reasons rather than frantically trying to burn off calories from unhealthy, unnecessary eating.

Q Can I stick to the Yoga for Weight Loss routine even though I am pregnant?

A If you are already on an exercise programme, fine, but get your midwife or doctor to give you the go-ahead. Be very gentle with the stretches, and do not do the inverted posture. Instead lie with your legs up against the wall or a chair, and your body on the floor.

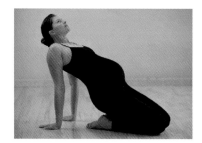

Q You say this is a de-addiction programme. Can you say more?

A When I first started practising yoga at the age of 29, I smoked cigarettes. The more I practised yoga, the more I felt good, and I started to be aware that when I was smoking I was detracting from all the wonderful benefits yoga was producing. So I chose to concentrate more on the benefits, and my desire for cigarettes just fell away. I had 'tasted' the joy, peace, and harmony that yoga brought and I wanted more of that and less of the false high that cigarettes can bring. Likewise, as you become more positive as a result of the Yoga for Weight Loss programme, your desire for a quickfood fix will lessen. I found this, and you definitely will, too, believe me.

Q Is yoga a religion?

A Yoga is about spirituality, rather than being a religion. People from many different religions find yoga a helpful way to connect more deeply with their own religious beliefs. On the other hand, you can have no belief and still find yoga beneficial. Yoga for Weight Loss helps connect you to your true, authentic self. I use terms that do not offend and give students the option to change, adapt or extract what they want.

Q Is Yoga for Weight Loss based on Hatha Yoga?

A Partly. Hatha Yoga is a type of yoga based on postures designed to make your body fit and healthy, so that you can aspire (if you want to, of course) to 'higher' things. In Sanskrit, the ancient language in which yoga was first documented, *ha* is the sun and *tha* the moon. It is symbolic of the fact that the sun and moon, *yang* and *yin*, or male and female, within each person need to be balanced for optimum health. As a step toward greater personal development, it can be useful to acknowledge both your male and female aspects. Be careful how you interpret this, however. I recall talking to one brave, lone male student in my class and telling him not to worry because I was half-man also, so to speak. I never saw him again!

Q Can I practise Yoga for Weight Loss from a book?

A Of course! All the information and motivation that you need is here in this book. However, nothing can replace the expertise and support that a trained yoga teacher can give you; also, the weekly class attendance is highly motivating and will keep you on track. You can check my website (see page 140) for an Accredited Yoga for Weight Loss teacher. Find one with whom you resonate and you will have discovered a little pot of gold.

Q What is a yoga guru, and are you one?

A The word 'guru' means 'dispeller of darkness'. Historically, a teacher of yoga would live in an *ashram*, which is basically a place of retreat from the world, dedicate their life to a yogic path, and be known as a 'guru'. A person who adopted the yogic path (a *sadhu*) would need to spend time in an *ashram* and be with their guru to 'see the light'. However, we live in a modern world where for most people this would be impractical or impossible, so if guru means 'dispeller of darkness', I'm sure we can all think of many people who shine a light for others in everyday terms. Think about it. Our partners, for instance. In fact all relationships have potential to provide 'growth moments' if we choose to be open to them. I do not see myself as a leading yogic master; I am just here to do my work. I often say that when we are working together, there is only one of us. So I am here for you, and you are here for me.

Q I have a bad back; can I still do the programme?

A It depends on what the problem is, but it pays to be careful. Get it checked out, and if your doctor or osteopath/chiropractor tells you you can go ahead, then do so. Proceed with caution. A good

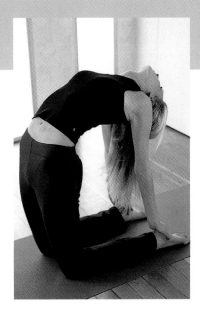

general rule is, if you feel pain — stop, and if in doubt — don't! Many practitioners prescribe yoga as an aid to recovery and prevention of further problems.

Q Do I have to stop eating meat and be a strict vegetarian to practise Yoga for Weight Loss?

A You do not have to impose any strict eating restrictions on yourself to follow my Yoga for Weight Loss programme. Some yogis eat meat, some do not. Most do not, because what tends to happen is that as you practise yoga regularly, your desire to eat meat will naturally diminish. Some of the great yogic masters say we should pay as much attention to what comes out of our mouths as to what we put in. You will enjoy the vitality and calmness that come from eating a simple, wholesome diet, and this might, or might not, include meat.

Q What about cigarettes? Do I need to give them up on this programme?

A When I first took up yoga, I smoked, but as I continued with the breathing exercises I started to realise that cigarettes were just negating all the effort and time I had put in to my practice. Eventually the desire for clean lungs, pure breath, fresh-smelling clothes and a longer, healthier life became more important than the quick high I got from a cigarette.

Q I like the occasional drink and can't get through the morning without my coffee fix. Surely in moderation they are OK?

A Moderation is definitely the best way, unless you particularly want to go down the hard path of giving everything up at once. I suggest just taking it easy and cutting down gradually, because as you practise your yoga, the desire for stimulants will effortlessly fall away. Yoga is a calming discipline, and anything stimulating does not really fit well with it, but you must make up your own mind. Certainly tea and coffee can make you jittery because of the caffeine in them, so do try to reduce your intake to one a day, and then try a coffee substitute such as Bambu or Barleycup, both of which are readily available from health food stores. If you wish, mix some

coffee with the substitute to start with, then gradually decrease the proportion of coffee. Similarly with alcohol: have a drink occasionally but remember that too much drinking is hazardous to your health. I believe that eventually you will find that the high from the yoga and your reconnection with the magnificence of your true self are so much better than the false high from alcohol.

Q Can yoga help your sex life?

A Of course — why do you think I like yoga so much?! Joking aside, Yoga for Weight Loss will not only help you lose weight and gain confidence, vitality and a sense of your inner beauty, but also bring about a reconnection with your inner self. This opens up your heart, so you can then approach your sex life with a new-found intimacy which will lead to the most beautiful, sensual sexual experiences. You make love with your body, mind and spirit — not just your body.

Q How soon should I expect results?

A You will gain benefits from the first day. People often comment after their first yoga class that they have had their best night's sleep ever. So from the first session, you will be calmer and happier, sleep better and generally feel that

everyone around you is less stressed – this is because *you* are less stressed! However, four weeks of determined, regular practice will produce a healthier, slimmer body, and you will look at life from a more positive perspective. These changes will be permanent and will enhance your life and make your relationships happier; but most of all the relationship you have with yourself will be enriched beyond your dreams.

Q Do you recommend fasting?

A I have found it very helpful. I recommend that you fast in a group, or one-to-one with a qualified practitioner, away from your own home. I also find that one day a week on fruit only is a good thing for my body, but only when I am living in a hot climate — it does not work for me in Scotland! After fasting, expect to feel clear-minded, rejuvenated and full of energy and a tremendous sense of positivity and empowerment. After I'd done one particular fast in California my mum asked if I'd had a face-lift!

Q Sometimes I just automatically put food in my mouth, and I don't know why. I don't even want it. I feel awful afterwards. Why do I do this?

A Often the way we eat is ruled by old habits or by our emotions. This often means that we use food as a temporary 'stuffing' of feelings. The underlying issue itself needs to be resolved before permanent relief can be found. Yoga can give you the awareness to discover whether your challenge is a habit or an emotional lack. Once you have that awareness, you can use the discipline of yoga to change that habit through some of the suggestions I have made in the book. If the cause is emotional, yoga can help you to develop the awareness to discover what is lacking, so that you can then devise a plan of action to fill the void or need in another way.

Q At what age do you recommend starting Yoga for Weight Loss?

A Yoga for Weight Loss is suitable for all ages.

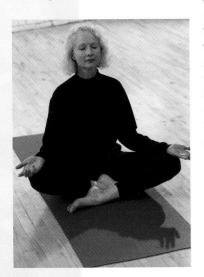

Q Sometimes my tummy bloats up and I look 6 months' pregnant. I'm not fat, but I really feel it. I look after myself otherwise. Why is this?

A You firstly need to check with your doctor that it is nothing to worry about. My hunch is that you have developed a food intolerance. You can check this at the doctor's with a blood test or by yourself with an exclusion diet. You do this by going without the suspected substance for two weeks, and then you do a pulse test. This involves taking your resting pulse rate. You do this by finding a pulse in your neck using a light touch of the middle three fingertips of your left hand to the right side of your neck. Be very gentle, and use a light touch. In your neck you will find the pulse on the side of the windpipe (alternatively, you can find it on the thumb side of your wrist just below where a watch strap would be). Eat some of your suspected food, then retake your pulse after 10, 30 and 60 minutes. If it rises by more than 10 points, you have a food intolerance. Don't despair, as there are many good substitutes on the market nowadays. Many people do have intolerances, the most common being wheat, dairy products, yeast, alcohol, coffee, tea, eggs, nuts and oranges. You, of course, can watch your own reactions to them. Personally, I find that stock cubes

make my eyelids swell, which I think must be something to do with the salt in them. Sometimes food intolerances can be temporary, and by eliminating the culprit food for a period you can then eat it in moderate amounts.

Q Organic food is so expensive, I just can't afford it. Can I do the programme anyway?

A Yes. You will still achieve good results. The whole programme is aimed at bringing your body fairly quickly back to a healthy point of balance where it then can digest and burn fat at the best rate for you. If you don't eat organic, it just might take a little longer. At first, compared to ordinary food, organic does seem a lot more expensive, but there are ways around this. Firstly, try to grow your own, even if it is just herbs or lettuce in a window box or tub. Make friends with someone who has a large garden and will sell or give you their surplus organic vegetables. Get to know when your local supermarket sells off its organic vegetables and chicken, and be there first! In some areas there are organic societies you can join. Their offers vary, but typically, if you commit for a year, you will get a box of organic vegetables delivered to a central point for you to pick up each week.

Points to Ponder

Sometimes stretching ourselves psychologically involves going out on a limb — but that is where the fruit is. If you would like to go just that bit farther or deeper with Yoga for Weight Loss, then think about these points and how they might relate to you. Take them one by one, and just spend some time really thinking about what they mean to you — you will be surprised at how much it can help.

Surrender to life's intelligence.

Watch nature. It doesn't need diets or instruction books in order to grow, produce flowers and seeds for the next cycle's growth. Maybe if we could tap into the universal life force through yoga we could know which foods are most beneficial for us, how much water to drink, what not to drink, and how to be generally more harmonious in living. I've certainly found this to be so; perhaps it would work for you, too.

Two words that will make you slim instantly — stop judging.

You feel fat because you compare yourself with others, whether friends or movie stars.

What you resist persists, what you accept dissolves.

Accepting yourself as you are does not mean inaction — it means not wasting time justifying how you got to where you are now.

You are as young as your spine.

This is why in yoga we devote a lot of time to spinal movement, as the spine is the highway of the body, where many of our body's energies and regulatory systems are transported.

What the mind can conceive (the new slim vibrant you), the body can achieve.

This is why Yoga for Weight Loss works from the inside out.

Don't put pressure on yourself.

Yoga for Weight Loss is about relieving tension and being drawn to weight loss naturally, rather than striving toward it.

Chutes and ladders

Life often seems like this: two steps forward and three back! However, often the backward moves help prepare us for the forward moves, and our greatest growth often takes place when we feel we are getting nowhere.

Eat to live not live to eat

As you follow your yoga programme you will naturally enjoy eating smaller portions.

The most difficult journey in the world is just over 30cm long; it is the journey from the head to the heart

That is, rather than using your mind all the time where logic rules, you start to act from your heart and take a more loving approach to life.

The mind is like the water of a lake

When the water is troubled it cannot reflect a clear image. The light that falls on it is distorted and produces a mosaic of colours that does not make sense. But if the water is calm, it reflects the sky and everything else as a perfect mirror. The mind, too, cannot 'reflect' truth if it is troubled by distraction and anxiety.

Fat mind

On those days when you wake up feeling larger than normal, don't say, 'I feel fat today;' instead say, 'I've got fat thoughts today.' This is more truthful.

And finally, some more sound bites, the slimming food for thought:

■ A lie we have about ourselves becomes our truth if it remains unchallenged.

■ Challenge yourself to be the best you can be. There is no failure – only not bothering to have a go.

■ There is strength in vulnerability.

■ Everything that gets worse with age gets better with yoga.

■ I don't have time NOT to exercise.

■ Nothing tastes as good as being slim feels.

■ It is the continual effort to be something other than what we really are that is the cause of all our problems.

■ You get what you expect and believe you will get.

■ The more you hate something, the more bound you are to it, and the more you love it, the freer you are.

■ Your outer world is a symbolic representation of that which is within you.

Resources

CELIA HAWE

Retreats, Talks/Seminars, Teacher Training: www.yogaforslimmers.com

Weight Loss Life Coaching: www.weightlosscoachingsupport.com

Life Coaching Skills Training, and Personal and Business Coaching: www.diamondcoaching.com

For your 28-day detox and eating programme

The Food Doctor's 'Cleanse' detox fruit and seed bar – highly recommended!
www.thefooddoctor.com

Dr Gillian McKeith's Living Food Energy Bar
info@mckeithresearch.com
www.drgillianmckeigh.com

Seasoning:
Bragg's Liquid Aminos
(plus information on healthy eating and cleansing regimes)
www.bragg.com

Grains of Desire grinder by the Cape Herb and Spice Company, distributed by Cavive Trading Ltd
50 Bell Crescent,
Westlake Business Park
Tokai, Cape Town, South Africa
www.capeherb.com

Marigold Swiss Vegetable Bouillon Powder (an instant broth based on vegetables and sea salt)
Marigold Foods, 102 Camley Street,
London NW1 0PF
Tel: 00 44 (0)20 7388 4515

Organic dried herbs grinder by Fiddes Payne (Herbs and Spices) Ltd
Pepper Alley, 3b Thorpe Way,
Banbury, Oxon. OX16 8XL
www.fiddespayne.co.uk

Vitasoy Creamy Original
Soya milk can take some getting used to! This is my favourite.
www.vitasoy.com

Food intolerance testing

Blood tests for food intolerances
York Nutritional Laboratory
Murton Way, Osbaldwick,
York YO19 5US
ynl@allergy.co.uk
www.allergy.co.uk

Nutrition

British Nutrition Foundation
www.nutrition.org.uk

Higher Nature Ltd
The Nutrition Centre, Burwash
Common, East Sussex N19 7LX
www.highernature.co.uk

Organic produce

The Soil Association
Bristol House, 40–56 Victoria Street,
Bristol BS1 6BY
www.soilassociation.org
This produces a directory of 450 outlets supplying organic produce, such as vegetables, meat, baby food, beer, wine, dairy produce, bread, cereals and specialities.

Phoenix Community Store
Tel: 00 44 (0)1309 690 110
www.findhorn.org/store
UK organic food retailer of the year which stocks an excellent selection of health food and products.

Veganism and Vegetarianism

Living and Raw Foods
www.living-foods.com
A site dedicated to providing comprehensive information on vegetarian food as well as recipes.

Vege Life
www.vegelife.com
A discussion forum site which is accompanied by press articles, recipes and an online shopping mall.

Vegetarian Resource Group
www.vrg.org
This site will give advice and explain everything about being a vegetarian.

Vegan Society
www.vegansociety.com
Find out all you need to know about a vegan lifestyle.

Tarla Dalal
www.tarladalal.com
A good source of vegetarian recipes from around the world, complete with a handy shopping list compiler.

Quorn
www.quorn.com
The healthy alternative to meat

Sprouters

Simply Nature
Old Factory Buildings, Battenhurst Road, Stonegate TN5 7DU
Tel: 00 44 (0)1580 201697
www.simply-nature.co.uk
Wheat-grass sprouters and natural products

Retreats and personal development

Findhorn Foundation Community
Tel: 00 44 (0)1309 690 311
www.findhorn.org
World-famous community for personal and spiritual development

Cortijo Romero
www.cortijo-romero.co.uk
Alternative holidays in southern Spain

Skyros
Tel: 00 44 (0)20 7284 3065
Alternative holidays in Greece

Coach University
www.coachu.com
Life coach training, or to find a life coach

International Coach Federation
www.coachfederation.org

Yoga classes and training

British Wheel of Yoga
1 Hamilton Place, Boston Road, Sleaford, Lincolnshire NG34 7ES
Tel: 00 44 (0)1529 306851
www.bwy.org.uk
This is where I did my yoga training and I highly recommend it. They hold courses and have books and videos for sale. You can also find out about BWY teachers in your area if you wish to supplement the programme in this book with other yoga classes.

Scottish Yoga Teachers Association
26 Brucehaven Road, Limekilns, Fife KY11 3HZ
Tel: 00 44 (0)1383 872825
www.yogascotland.org.uk

The World of Yoga
www.yoyoga.com
This yoga site promotes a holistic approach to getting in shape, and includes recipes and thoughts on yoga philosophy.

Yoga Site
www.yogasite.com
This site takes a hands-on approach to exercise and offers instruction on postures as well as links to other yoga sites.

Yoga Place E2
1st Floor, 449–453 Bethnal Green
Road, London E2 9QH
Tel: 00 44 (0)20 7739 5195
www.yogaplace.co.uk
For courses and workshops

Clothing and equipment

Yoga Matters
www.yogamatters.com
Sells yoga products

The Yoga Shop
www.theyogashop.co.uk
Sell yoga clothes, mats, cards,
charts and herbs

Asquith Ltd
Tel: 00 44 (0)20 7792 8909
www.asquith.ltd.uk
Exclusive yoga clothing. Contact the
above for stockists and mail order.

Casall/Viva UK Ltd
2 Market Place, Somerton,
Somerset TA11 7LX
Tel: 00 44 (0)1458 273 394
www.casall.com
General sportswear company

Further reading

Weight watchers' cookbooks
contain great recipes, and there are
also recipes on their website,
www.weightwatchers.com.
Rosemary Conley's books are also a
good investment, since they contain
recipes for tasty low-fat dishes.

Health & Fitness Magazine online
www.hfonline.co.uk

**How to Know God: The Yoga
Aphorisms of Patanjali**
Translated by Swami
Prabhavananda and
Christopher Isherwood
A wonderful little book that
says it all

Kindred Spirit Magazine
Foxhole, Dartington, Devon TQ9 6EB
Tel: 00 44 (0)1803 866686
mailorder@kindredspirit.co.uk
www.kindredspirit.co.uk

Loving What Is
Byron Katie
A book to help make sense of any
blame regarding weight issues as
well as a host of other life issues
www.thework.org

Staying Healthy with Nutrition
Elson M. Haas, M.D.
A huge book but very educational
and helpful

Yoga and Health Magazine
www.yogaandhealthmag.co.uk

Your Body's Many Cries for Water
Dr F. Batmanghelidj

The Yoga Cookbook
Recipes from the Sivananda Yoga
Vedanta Centre. www.sivananda.org

Yoga for the West
Ian Rawlinson

Yoga Journal
Quarterly, with lots of contacts,
products and interesting articles
www.yogajournal.com

Yoga Magazine
Mind, Body, Spirit
26 York Street
London W1U 6PZ
info@yogamagazine.co.uk
www.yogamagazine.co.uk

Yoga the Iyengar Way
Silva Mehta and Shyam Mehta

Yoga: the Path to Holistic Health
B.K.S. Iyengar

The Postures:
A Quick-reference Guide

As you work your way through the programme, you may find it useful to refer to this list of exercises and postures, so you can find them quickly. Complete each posture at least once, holding for 4–7 breaths. Do it every day – religiously!

Index